W9-AYN-443

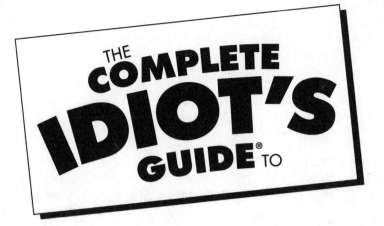

THE COMPLETE IDIOT'S GUIDE® TO

Eating Clean

PORTER COUNTY PUBLIC LIBRARY

Hebron Public Library
201 W. Sigler Street
Hebron, IN 46341

by Diane A. Welland, M.S., R.D.

NF   641.5637 WEL   HEB
Welland, Diane.
The complete idiot's guide to
33410010698225   JAN 28 2010

PORTER COUNTY LIBRARY SYSTEM

DISCARD

ALPHA

A member of Penguin Group (USA) Inc.

This book is dedicated to my husband Kevin—chef extraordinaire, recipe tester, and always-willing taster. Thank you.

ALPHA BOOKS

Published by the Penguin Group

Penguin Group (USA) Inc., 375 Hudson Street, New York, New York 10014, USA

Penguin Group (Canada), 90 Eglinton Avenue East, Suite 700, Toronto, Ontario M4P 2Y3, Canada (a division of Pearson Penguin Canada Inc.)

Penguin Books Ltd., 80 Strand, London WC2R 0RL, England

Penguin Ireland, 25 St. Stephen's Green, Dublin 2, Ireland (a division of Penguin Books Ltd.)

Penguin Group (Australia), 250 Camberwell Road, Camberwell, Victoria 3124, Australia (a division of Pearson Australia Group Pty. Ltd.)

Penguin Books India Pvt. Ltd., 11 Community Centre, Panchsheel Park, New Delhi—110 017, India

Penguin Group (NZ), 67 Apollo Drive, Rosedale, North Shore, Auckland 1311, New Zealand (a division of Pearson New Zealand Ltd.)

Penguin Books (South Africa) (Pty.) Ltd., 24 Sturdee Avenue, Rosebank, Johannesburg 2196, South Africa

Penguin Books Ltd., Registered Offices: 80 Strand, London WC2R 0RL, England

Copyright © 2009 by Diane A. Welland

All rights reserved. No part of this book shall be reproduced, stored in a retrieval system, or transmitted by any means, electronic, mechanical, photocopying, recording, or otherwise, without written permission from the publisher. No patent liability is assumed with respect to the use of the information contained herein. Although every precaution has been taken in the preparation of this book, the publisher and author assume no responsibility for errors or omissions. Neither is any liability assumed for damages resulting from the use of information contained herein. For information, address Alpha Books, 800 East 96th Street, Indianapolis, IN 46240.

THE COMPLETE IDIOT'S GUIDE TO and Design are registered trademarks of Penguin Group (USA) Inc.

International Standard Book Number: 978-1-59257-946-4
Library of Congress Catalog Card Number: 2009928401

11   10   09   8   7   6   5   4   3   2   1

Interpretation of the printing code: The rightmost number of the first series of numbers is the year of the book's printing; the rightmost number of the second series of numbers is the number of the book's printing. For example, a printing code of 09-1 shows that the first printing occurred in 2009.

Printed in the United States of America

Note: This publication contains the opinions and ideas of its author. It is intended to provide helpful and informative material on the subject matter covered. It is sold with the understanding that the author and publisher are not engaged in rendering professional services in the book. If the reader requires personal assistance or advice, a competent professional should be consulted.

The author and publisher specifically disclaim any responsibility for any liability, loss, or risk, personal or otherwise, which is incurred as a consequence, directly or indirectly, of the use and application of any of the contents of this book.

Most Alpha books are available at special quantity discounts for bulk purchases for sales promotions, premiums, fundraising, or educational use. Special books, or book excerpts, can also be created to fit specific needs.

For details, write: Special Markets, Alpha Books, 375 Hudson Street, New York, NY 10014.

Publisher: *Marie Butler-Knight*
Editorial Director: *Mike Sanders*
Senior Managing Editor: *Billy Fields*
Acquisitions Editor: *Tom Stevens*
Development Editor: *Jennifer Moore*
Senior Production Editor: *Megan Douglass*
Copy Editor: *Emily Garner*

Cartoonist: *Steve Barr*
Cover Designer: *Rebecca Batchelor*
Book Designer: *Trina Wurst*
Indexer: *Johnna VanHoose Dinse*
Layout: *Ayanna Lacey*
Proofreader: *Laura Caddell*

Contents at a Glance

Contents

Appendixes

Introduction

Eating clean is more than just a diet. It's a healthy approach to eating that emphasizes whole, unprocessed, and unrefined foods.

For many people, weight loss is the main attraction to the clean eating lifestyle. It's easy to shed pounds and build lean muscle mass when you're not eating gobs of refined fats, sugars, and carbohydrates and you're working out regularly. Others want improved health and increased energy—two other benefits of eating clean. Last but not least is the fact that many people are just tired of eating highly processed foods with artificial ingredients and additives they can't even pronounce. This yearning for simple, wholesome food that's prepared with natural, healthful ingredients is the reason eating clean is becoming so popular.

Unfortunately, many people are so dependent on salty, sugary, and refined convenience foods they don't even know how to start. This book shows you what to do, from taking little steps like choosing water over soda or brown rice instead of white rice to making a clean sweep of it by purging your pantry, refrigerator, and freezer of processed foods. All the tools and techniques you need to clean up your diet—including shopping tips and restaurant strategies—are in the following pages.

Most important is the fact that once you understand why and how to clean up your diet and get healthy, you'll find dozens of recipes and cooking techniques for putting clean eating principles into practice. I've included recipes for a wealth of breakfast foods, drinks, snacks, meals, and desserts—all clean, all natural, and all delicious—that demonstrate just how incredibly flavorful, easy, and satisfying clean eating can be.

Turn the pages to discover the amazing health benefits of a nutritious, unprocessed, unrefined diet. Prepare to be impressed!

How This Book Is Organized

This book is divided into six parts. Each part addresses a different aspect of eating clean.

Part 1, "The ABCs of Being Clean," provides you with everything you need to know about going clean. It explains what clean eating means and why this style of eating is good for your health. It also discusses the seven basic principles of eating clean and how you can turn these principles into action. Learn how to manage your time in the kitchen, be a savvy shopper, and dine out smart. Explore some of the challenges clean eaters face and strategies to overcome them. Finally, learn what it means to be clean and green, and clean and wheat-free and dairy-free.

Part 2, "Jump-Start Your Morning," introduces you to clean breakfasts including hot and cold cereals, egg dishes, pancakes, and baked muffins and breads. Here is everything you need to face the morning with a smile.

Since snacks are an important part of eating clean, they deserve their own section. **Part 3, "Light Bites,"** covers all types of clean snacks—from substantial grab-and-go finger foods and fruit salads to fruity salsas, sauces, and jams. You'll also find drink recipes featuring teas, milk, and juice.

Part 4, "Lovely Lunches," presents you with a variety of interesting, unusual, and wonderfully delectable lunch options that run the gamut from soups and salads to sandwiches.

Part 5, "Dinner Designs," does more than give you recipes for dozens of outstanding clean dinner entrées. This part also covers techniques for managing scratch cooking, such as ideas for 30-minute meals, techniques for cooking two meals in one, and preparing large batches of long-cooking foods to pull out when you need them. Also included is an array of vegetable sides and starches, plus clean condiments, sauces, and marinades that are sure to add some spice to your life.

Part 6, "Sweet Endings," tempts your taste buds with wonderfully clean desserts, including creams, parfaits, crisps, and puddings. These dreamy endings get most of their sweetness naturally from fruit. You'll also find recipes for clean cakes and cookies, using all whole grain flours and unrefined processed sugar. Who said clean eating isn't fun!

In the back of the book are appendixes where you'll find helpful information on your way to exploring clean eating. This includes a five-day menu plan, which shows you how to follow a clean eating diet pattern of six small meals a day, and a glossary defining any terms you might not be familiar with.

Extras

In every chapter you'll find these boxes that share important information you should know about the clean eating lifestyle, particular recipes, or specific foods.

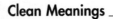 **Clean Meanings** _____

Turn to these boxes for definitions of words or phrases you might not be familiar with.

 Clean Cuts _____

These boxes offer tips and tricks to make your life easier in the kitchen.

Dirty Secrets _____

Eating clean poses certain challenges, and these boxes help you overcome them by pointing out foods to steer clear of.

Wholesome Habits _____

Here you'll find enlightening insights about food, culinary arts, and living a healthy lifestyle.

Acknowledgments

I would like to express my heartfelt thanks to all the people who have helped make this book possible: especially Marilyn Allen of Allen O'Shea Agency for having blind faith in me; all the staff at Alpha Books especially Tom Stevens, Jennifer Moore, Megan Douglass, and Emily Garner; everyone who answered my endless questions, including Susan Male Smith, Sheila Weiss, Roberta Dyuff, Cynthia Harriman, and Dean Edelman; Janet Sass for her great insights and discriminating palate, and all the dietitian colleagues who supported and encouraged me.

I would also like to thank my gracious family for bearing with me through countless hours of research, typing, and cooking. This includes my ever-patient husband Kevin, and my children: Leslie, chief dish-dryer and baby-sitter; Christopher, for helping out when I needed him and tasting most of the dishes; and Sophia, for always giving me a hug when I needed it. Without their help and support this book would not have been possible.

Special Thanks to the Technical Reviewer

The Complete Idiot's Guide to Eating Clean was reviewed by an expert who double-checked the accuracy of what you'll learn here, to help us ensure that this book gives you everything you need to know about eating clean. Special thanks are extended to Alexandra Hart Bosshart, who has been a friend and a colleague for many years. Her insights and culinary knowledge are appreciated.

Trademarks

All terms mentioned in this book that are known to be or are suspected of being trademarks or service marks have been appropriately capitalized. Alpha Books and Penguin Group (USA) Inc. cannot attest to the accuracy of this information. Use of a term in this book should not be regarded as affecting the validity of any trademark or service mark.

Part 1

The ABCs of Being Clean

Eating clean is more than just a diet—it's a lifestyle with an overall focus on sound nutrition, good health, and regular physical activity. Since clean food is typically low in fat, calories, sodium, and sugar (all the bad stuff!) and high in fiber, vitamins, and minerals (all the good stuff!), clean eaters enjoy incredible health benefits like weight loss, reduced risk of chronic illness, and improved strength.

Living clean in a dirty world takes some adjustments. You'll learn to choose whole natural foods over refined, processed foods in the kitchen, at the grocery store, and when dining out. You'll also get simple but powerful tips for keeping clean and healthy.

Finally, we'll introduce you to a clean green lifestyle, explaining how to choose organic, locally grown, whole foods over conventional ones. And for some people, being clean also means removing all wheat and/or dairy products from their diet, so we've covered that, too.

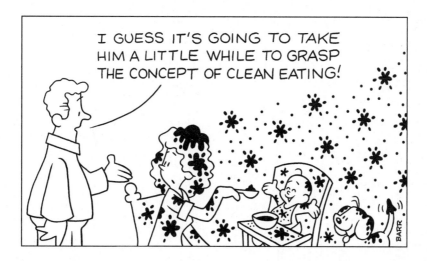

A Case for Eating Clean

In This Chapter

- ◆ What eating clean is all about
- ◆ Tracing the history of clean eating
- ◆ Eating clean to stay lean
- ◆ Optimizing your health

Clean eating is all about eating healthful, high-quality, nutritious food. But as any clean eater will tell you, it's more than just a diet. It's a lifestyle—a sound approach to eating and living well that maximizes your energy and optimizes your health. Losing weight is probably the main reason most people start eating clean, and rightly so.

Eating clean enables you to shed pounds and build lean muscle mass without skipping a meal or ever being hungry. But clean eaters experience other health benefits, too, like better blood sugar control, lower blood pressure, lower cholesterol, and reduced risk of many common chronic illnesses. We also sleep better, handle stress better, and have overall better health than people eating a standard American diet. In this chapter, we'll share the scientific and nutritional theories behind these health benefits.

Although the term *clean eating* is relatively new, the principles of emphasizing whole, unrefined foods; grazing on small meals throughout the day; and trimming fat, sugar, and calories have been around for decades. The clean eating philosophy has its roots in the natural health foods movement of the 1960s, which shunned processed foods. At the time, the diet was as much about rebelling against "the establishment" and finding one's own individuality as it was about health and nutrition. Taste sometimes took a back seat, but the diet stuck. Now it's being adopted by regular people who are interested in living a healthy, happy life.

What Is Eating Clean?

Clean eating is a diet that focuses on eating whole, natural foods that are not *processed*. This means they do not contain any man-made ingredients or unnecessary *food additives*.

Most processed or manufactured foods, like those that come out of a box, bag, or can, contain a large amount of man-made food additives. Purists cut out all processed foods—even store-bought bread, cheese, and juices—but for most of us, simply minimizing processed foods or avoiding only highly processed manufactured foods like frozen or boxed meals, fancy side dishes, and desserts is enough to make a difference in our diet and our health. (Food additives and processed foods will be covered more in depth in Chapter 2.)

Clean eating also means choosing unrefined over *refined foods*. Unrefined foods are in their natural state and include whole grains, whole grain flours, dried beans, legumes, and natural sweeteners like honey and maple syrup. Refined foods have been modified to make them easier to eat or digest and supply a concentrated source of calories, meaning it's easy to eat too much of them. They also generally have a longer shelf life than unrefined foods, which is why we like them so much. Unfortunately, refined foods often lose vital nutrients during processing.

SOAP | **Clean Meanings** _____

Processed foods are any foods that have been altered to change their physical, chemical, microbiological, or sensory properties.

Food additives are ingredients added to food to improve safety and freshness, nutritional value, taste, texture, or appearance. They can be natural or artificial.

Refined foods are foods that have their coarse or fibrous part removed, resulting in a loss of nutrients.

The two major refined foods in our diet are refined grains, such as white flour and white rice; and refined sugar, known as white, granulated, or table sugar. For most people, avoiding these refined foods is, at first, the hardest part of eating clean, but once you get used to it, you'll find whole unrefined foods like brown rice, whole grain breads, and whole wheat pastas are not only more tasty and nutritious than their refined counterparts but also more satisfying.

In addition, clean eating means eating meals that are naturally balanced and not loaded with saturated fat and calories. Cutting out the fat, sugar, and salt is actually easier than you think, particularly if you stick to natural unrefined foods over refined processed ones. Still, you can't go crazy and eat as much as you want, even when you're eating healthy food. Too many calories—no matter the source—will be stored as fat.

Portions are small, but this doesn't mean you have to go hungry. Clean eaters fill up frequently, eating every two to three hours and fitting in five to six meals every day. This includes three main meals—breakfast, lunch, and dinner—and two to three substantial snacks, composed of protein, carbohydrate, and some fat. Eating this way helps you avoid overeating and keeps your energy level constant throughout the day.

Finally, the clean eating lifestyle is an active one, with daily physical activity. Regular workouts are recommended at least five days a week.

In an ideal world we would eat clean all of the time and exercise every day. But for most of us this isn't realistic. Certainly, the closer you follow this lifestyle the more benefits you will reap, but even small steps like buying whole wheat bread instead of white or switching from white rice to brown can make a difference.

Many people start small and then gradually grow into the lifestyle over time. To enjoy maximum benefits from a clean eating lifestyle, we encourage you to strive for a diet that's 75 to 80 percent clean and to maintain a regular exercise routine. Ultimately, it's a personal decision. For some people, going 50 percent processed-free is enough to keep them slim, trim, happy, and healthy. Others simply eliminate all processed meals like frozen and boxed dinners. Choose what works for you.

Wholesome Habits

Some people believe clean eating is more than just removing processed and refined foods. They seek out only organic and naturally-raised food, excluding anything grown or raised with synthetic pesticides, fertilizers, and hormones. For others clean eating encompasses being wheat-free and dairy-free. I'll talk more about both of these variations on the clean eating diet in Chapter 5.

Why Pass on Processed?

So, what's the matter with processed foods? Fat, sugar, salt, chemicals, and calories—most processed foods contain loads of them. For this reason they're usually the first to go when people are trying to lose weight, improve their health, or simply overhaul their eating habits. Here's what clean eating can do for you.

Stay Clean, Stay Lean

Many people who go clean lose weight without even trying. Those who do try find that the weight comes off easily. That's because clean eaters avoid the two main weight gain culprits—refined sugars and refined flours, which contain lots of calories and little nutrition. Because starchy foods and sweets don't fill you up, many people eat way too much of them in an attempt to satisfy their hunger.

Honing in on whole fruits, vegetables, beans, and whole grains instead of processed foods also means you're getting plenty of fiber. Your body digests high-fiber foods more slowly than sugary, starchy foods, which means you'll feel full longer. As an added bonus, foods high in fiber tend to be lower in calories and higher in valuable vitamins and minerals. Studies show that people who lose weight eating whole grains have smaller waists—meaning they lose more of their excess pounds around the abdominal area—than those who don't fill up on fiber.

> **Dirty Secrets**
>
> Studies show people who eat a diet high in refined and processed foods tend to put on weight around the middle. This belly fat is not only harder to lose than weight in the legs and thighs; it also increases your risk for heart disease, stroke, diabetes, and dementia such as Alzheimer's disease.

Watching your fat intake is another aspect of eating clean. Here the focus is on natural, minimally processed, and unprocessed fats like olive oil, peanut oil, avocados, and olives, and staying away from foods high in unhealthy saturated and man-made trans fats.

Saturated fats raise cholesterol and increase your risk of heart disease. They are naturally found in the fat of meat, poultry, milk, cheese, eggs, and other dairy products. In the vegetable kingdom, they're in coconut and palm oil.

Trans fats are most prevalent in the food supply as man-made fats created by adding hydrogen to liquid fats and turning them into a solid or semisolid form. On labels they are listed as "hydrogenated" or "partially hydrogenated" fats. Today, they are considered worse than saturated fats for increasing risk of heart disease. Look for a total ban on trans fats in manufactured foods in the near future.

The final weapon in the clean eaters' weight loss arsenal is protein. Some type of protein is eaten at every meal and snack. Protein is essential for myriad functions in the body, but is especially important for building and maintaining lean muscle, which naturally burns more calories than body fat. In addition, eating high-protein foods can actually curb your appetite and thus help reduce your caloric intake. Though scientists don't yet know why this is the case, they do know protein makes you feel fuller and more satisfied than starchy carbohydrates and maybe even fat.

It's important to keep in mind that to optimize weight loss, these dietary changes must be paired with daily physical activity. Being active not only burns more calories but it keeps you from eating. Combine clean eating with daily exercise and you will be shedding pounds and looking good in no time.

> **Wholesome Habits**
>
> Next time you want something to nosh on, try grabbing a handful of nuts. Although high in fat (albeit the good kind), nuts are also rich in plant protein, fiber, vitamin E, and minerals like magnesium and copper. Nuts have been found to make you feel fuller longer and several studies show eating one small handful of nuts every day can actually help dieters lose weight.

Curbing Chronic Illness

The top three leading causes of death in the United States—heart disease, cancer, and stroke—are directly influenced by diet. Obesity is growing to epidemic proportions, and the Centers for Disease Control reports new diabetes cases are up 90 percent from 1995. Many health organizations, including the American Heart Association, the American Diabetes Association, and the American Medical Association, believe that poor diet and sedentary lifestyles are to blame for much of these problems.

Nutrition research links diets low in fiber and high in fat, saturated fat, sodium, and simple sugars to today's most common chronic illnesses. In contrast, clean eating is high in fiber—loaded with fruits, vegetables, and whole grains—and low in fat, saturated fat, sodium, and sugar. In other words, a clean diet is very much in line with what major health organizations recommend we should be eating. Not only will this way of eating help you look and feel better, it can also reduce your risk of heart disease, cancer, diabetes, stroke, and other obesity-related illnesses. The payoff is a longer, healthier life.

Heart Health

Aside from not smoking, the American Heart Association (AHA) says the best thing you can do to keep your ticker running smoothly is to eat a healthy diet and get regular exercise. This will reduce cholesterol, high blood pressure, and keep your weight in check. Heart healthy eating means choosing a diet loaded with nutrient-rich and high-fiber foods like fruits, vegetables, and beans; avoiding saturated and trans fats by eating lean meat, fish, and poultry; and cutting back on salt and sugar. Sound familiar? It should—these are the clean eating principles exactly.

Regular exercise is important for your heart, too. Recent research shows active women enjoy 18 percent lower rates of heart disease compared to their sedentary counterparts regardless of weight. Both obese and normal weight women were involved in the study.

Keeping Cancer at Bay

Like heart disease, certain cancers feed on rich, fatty, low-fiber diets. The World Health Organization says dietary factors account for about 30 percent of all cancers in Western countries. Cancers most closely related to diet are colon, breast, stomach, esophagus, mouth, endometrial, and ovarian cancer. Like the AHA, the American Institute of Cancer Research (AICR) recommends consuming a diet containing high-fiber fruits, vegetables, whole grains, and legumes; maintaining a healthy lean weight; and daily physical activity. The AICR also recommends avoiding sugary drinks and high-calorie processed foods high in added sugars or fat and low in nutrients, and limiting salty foods and processed meats like bacon and sausage.

Dirty Secrets _____

It is estimated that the average American adult consumes approximately 4,000 mg of sodium per day—much more than the 2,400 mg (or less) of sodium the U.S. Dietary Guidelines recommends we should be eating. One teaspoon of salt equals about 2,300 mg sodium.

Achieving a Healthy Blood Pressure

So, what's the matter with salt? Too much sodium leads to high blood pressure, also called hypertension. Over time, high blood pressure can lead to heart attack or stroke. What exactly is high blood pressure? A blood pressure reading of 140 over 90 or greater is considered high. The first, or top, number represents systolic blood pressure, which is the pressure of the heart on arteries when the heart contracts. The second, or bottom, number is diastolic blood pressure, a measure of the pressure of the heart at rest. Normal blood pressure is in the range of 120/80; anything between that and 140/90 is considered pre-hypertensive, or borderline. Most people with high blood pressure are salt sensitive, meaning if they decrease their salt, as well as lose weight and exercise, these numbers will drop.

Most of our salt comes from processed foods (I'll talk more about that in Chapter 2), and most people think salt equals flavor. Unfortunately, the more salt you eat the more you'll want because your taste buds become desensitized with repeated exposure. This is why many people who switch from a highly processed diet to a clean one initially think food tastes bland.

Dirty Secrets _____

Excess sodium also raises your risk for stomach cancer and kidney disease, and increases calcium losses, resulting in brittle bones.

Luckily, you can retrain your taste buds. All it takes is a little time and patience. Since most processed foods are eliminated on a clean eating regimen, salt intake is automatically low.

Better Blood Sugar Levels

Sugar—you can't live with it, and you can't live without it. Sugar, in the form of glucose, circulates in your blood and provides energy to fuel your cells. But too much sugar can wreak havoc on your system, causing you to gain weight, upsetting your natural blood sugar balance, and contributing to a slew of other health problems like heart and kidney disease.

Despite its drawbacks, people tend to love sugar. We were born to—it's in our genes. We also love starchy foods, which break down into sugars in the body. The problem is that most of the sugars and starches found in the typical American diet are highly refined, simple carbohydrates like high-fructose corn syrup, table sugar, and white flour. Your body absorbs these substances very quickly, causing your blood sugar levels to spike upward, then fall quickly. For the 23.6 million people who suffer from diabetes, a disease in which the body can't properly utilize its glucose, this can be a serious problem.

Dirty Secrets _____

Fifty-seven million Americans are estimated to have pre-diabetes, which means their glucose metabolism is impaired. Diabetes cases are skyrocketing, too. According to the Centers for Disease Control new diabetes cases are up 90 percent from just a decade ago.

Even if you don't have diabetes, eating too many refined simple sugars and starches and low fiber foods can still spell trouble. In addition to taxing your blood glucose system and expanding your waistline, it can raise your risk of getting diabetes in the first place. Overconsuming sugary drinks may also put you at risk of cardiovascular disease, by raising the amount of fats that circulate in your blood stream.

Natural sugars and unrefined starches found in fruits, vegetables, and whole grains don't have this effect on blood sugar and blood fat levels and are less likely to add waist weight, mainly because the fiber and protein in these foods are absorbed more slowly by the body; plus, they tend to have fewer calories. Eating small meals throughout the day, another clean eating virtue, also ensures you're getting the energy you need to keep you going. Perhaps that's the reason why clean eaters stay revved up throughout the day.

Battle the Bulge

The United States has one of the highest obesity rates in the world. One out of every three people are classified as obese. Although it's possible to be overweight, according to a height/weight chart, and still be lean (think of bodybuilders), that isn't usually the case for most people. It's also possible to have a body weight in the "desirable" or "normal" range and still be fat, if you have a high fat to lean ratio. Normal body fat for women is 25 to 30 percent, while for men it ranges from 18 to 23 percent.

Obesity is determined by body mass index or BMI. To find out your BMI, multiply your weight in pounds by 700, then divide the result by your height in inches, then divide that result by your height in inches a second time. This is your BMI. A BMI below 18.5 is underweight, 18.5 to 24.9 is a healthy weight, 25.0 to 29.9 is overweight, and over 30 is obese.

> **Wholesome Habits**
>
> Obesity is more prevalent in certain ethnic minority groups. Among those at higher risk are non-Hispanic black women and Mexican American women. The number of overweight children has also risen dramatically, nearly tripling over a 25 year-period from 1979 to 2004.

As your weight goes up, so does your chance of developing heart disease, diabetes, cancer, high blood pressure, high cholesterol, gout, and breathing and sleep disorders. This extra weight can even shorten your life, particularly those with BMIs over 40.

Managing your weight is simply a matter of calories in versus calories out. If you're overweight or obese you're taking in more calories than you're expending. To lose weight you need to burn more calories (exercise more) than you take in. Most people typically cut 500 calories a day, which leads to a

1 to 2 pound weight loss a week. By eating small meals throughout the day, it's easier to manage your hunger and stop yourself from overeating.

Build a Better Body

Many people switch to eating clean just to feel better and have more energy. Clean eaters have a reputation for vim and vigor, and a get-up-and-go mentality that's more than just attitude. The truth is clean eaters really do have more energy and feel less stressed than those following a typical American diet. Why? It's the lifestyle.

Diet is only part of the picture, but it's a big part. People who live on high-fat, calorie-laden processed foods are often tired, stressed out, and depressed. This type of food drags you down, leaving you bloated, overweight, and unhappy. Even if you do experience a spurt of energy (usually caused by excess sugar), it is generally short-lived, followed by an even lower drop in vitality. Clean eaters don't suffer from these ups and downs.

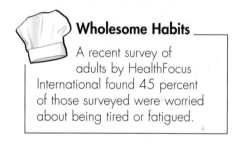

Wholesome Habits

A recent survey of adults by HealthFocus International found 45 percent of those surveyed were worried about being tired or fatigued.

Following a regular eating pattern and avoiding refined sugars and starches means you keep your engine revved up throughout the day. Balancing carbohydrates with fiber and protein prevents a boost in brain serotonin, a substance that makes you sleepy (serotonin rises when you eat primarily carbohydrates, like a big bowl of pasta marinara). At the same time, clean eaters also report fewer sleep problems and better mental health.

Keeping well-hydrated is another fatigue-buster—one clean eaters pay special attention to. Dehydration zaps energy by slowing down your body's metabolic rate. Water refuels your cells. You can get water in beverages like unsweetened tea and diluted juices, but you get plenty of water from fruits and vegetables, too.

Finally, clean eaters are active people. Exercising is the best stress-buster and fatigue fighter there is. It's also great for getting your mind off your problems and improving your mood. Physically, working out gets the blood pumping, improves circulation, builds strong bones and sexy muscles, plus it keeps your heart and lungs pumping more efficiently (more on this in Chapter 2).

The Least You Need to Know

- Clean eating focuses on whole fruits, vegetables, whole grains, and fresh meats, fish, and poultry while avoiding processed and refined foods.

- Today's lifestyle and food trends are perfectly suited to eating clean.

- Clean eating helps you stay lean and lose weight by focusing on lower calorie nutrient-rich foods and eliminating high-calorie processed foods.

- Eating clean can reduce the risk of many serious chronic illnesses like heart disease, cancer, stroke, high blood pressure, diabetes, and obesity.

- Following a clean lifestyle can improve your mental well-being.

Seven Simple Steps to Eating Clean

In This Chapter

- ◆ Basic principles of a clean eating lifestyle
- ◆ Favorite foods you can count on
- ◆ Why smaller meals are better
- ◆ Thirst-quenching clean drinks
- ◆ The importance of being active

Many of the basic principles of eating clean are similar to recommendations made by public health organizations like the U.S. Department of Agriculture, the American Heart Association, and the American Cancer Society. The guidelines are so close that when I'm asked to explain what eating clean is, I often see nods of recognition, followed by, "that's the way I try to eat" or "that's the way I eat already" or even "that's the way we should be eating." No surprises here. Most people know healthy diet concepts when they see them, it's just a matter of being motivated enough to actually follow through on them.

In this chapter we explain the seven guiding principles behind eating clean, give you an idea of some of the fabulous foods and drinks you should stock up on, and show you how to put this philosophy into practice. For those of you whose diet is already relatively clean, look at this chapter as a way to recharge your batteries, expand your culinary know-how, and fine-tune your food. For those of you who need a serious dietary overhaul, consider this chapter a way to kick-start the process. Think of these principles as goals to strive for, and take pride in every small step you make.

Eat a Whole Lot of Whole Foods

Whole foods in their most natural form are the backbone of eating clean. While fresh produce is an essential component of a clean diet, you don't have to be a vegetarian to eat clean. Fresh meat, fish, poultry, and game are also an important part of a clean eater's meal plan, as are whole grains and fresh dried beans.

Cooking and preparing delicious foods is simple as long as you keep a couple of things in mind.

First, choose wisely. Fresh foods are generally more fragile than processed or packaged foods, particularly if they have to travel long distances to get to you. That's because they don't have any preservatives or additives. This is especially true for meat, fish, poultry, produce, and dairy. At the store, be sure and check the "sell by" or "best used by date" if it has one. Then give it a good once over, making sure if it's wrapped the seal is not broken or leaking and, if it's produce, it's not too soft, too hard, moldy, or bruised.

Second, use it right away. Unlike processed or packaged foods, which can often last on the shelf for months, fresh foods go bad quickly. Don't buy more than you can eat in a sitting or two, unless you plan to freeze it. Eat your fresh food within two to three days.

This leads me to my third tip: handle your fresh foods with care. Most meat, produce, and dairy needs to be refrigerated immediately. Dry goods need to be stored in the pantry in a cool, dry place. While some dry goods do have a long shelf life, it is usually still shorter than refined, processed food.

Are You Dense?

Every food group has good and bad choices, and it isn't always obvious which is which. But, if you follow this simple rule you're sure to make your life a lot easier: always choose foods with maximum *nutrient density*.

High–nutrient density foods deliver the most nutritional bang for your buck with the fewest calories. For example, an apple loaded with fiber, vitamins, and minerals is more nutrient dense than a glass of apple juice, which is higher in sugar and calories. Compared to 1¹/₂ ounces of cheddar cheese, an 8 ounce glass of skim milk is the more nutrient dense. Although both contain the same amount of calcium, the skim milk has half the calories, not to mention zero fat.

Most nutrient dense foods—like fruits, vegetables, and legumes—are naturally low in calories, making them ideal choices when watching your weight and budgeting calories.

Low–nutrient density foods, on the other hand, are often pegged as *empty-calories* because they provide lots of energy and little else, lacking protein, vitamins, minerals, and fiber. In addition, almost all empty-calorie foods such as sodas, pastries, candy, potato chips, and other salty or sweet snacks are highly processed and refined.

SOAP | **Clean Meanings** _____

Nutrient density is a measure of the nutrient content compared to calorie levels. The more the nutrients and the fewer the calories, the higher the nutrient density. **Empty-calorie foods** are foods that are high in calories and very low in nutritive value. They are generally high in fat, salt, and sugar.

Count on Color

As you begin to build up your whole foods repertoire, you'll notice your meals will become more colorful. Colorful foods do more than just make your plate look beautiful and kick-start your appetite. They also promote good health.

When it comes to colorful fruits and vegetables, generally the more vivid the hue, the more beneficial phytochemicals they contain. Phytochemicals are plant compounds that give fruits, vegetables, beans, and grains their distinct characteristics. In the body, they are involved in a number of positive activities. Many phytochemicals are antioxidants.

Fruits, veggies, and legumes are naturally a good source of other antioxidants, too, like vitamins A, C, and E. Antioxidants protect the body from free radical damage. Free radicals are oxygen molecules that bounce around the body wreaking havoc. They speed up the body's aging process and increase risk of disease. Free radicals result from normal metabolism, stress, poor diet, pollutants, and other environmental insults. We are constantly under free radical attack. The more antioxidant-rich foods we eat the better.

As a general rule, choose deep, dark colored foods first, then complement them with a variety of brightly colored, vibrant-looking foods. The combination means you'll be sitting down to a rainbow of colors at every meal. To help you out, here is a list of colors (and foods) you should aim to eat on a regular basis:

- Dark green leafy vegetables like spinach, kale, and mustard greens
- Orange and yellow foods like pumpkin, sweet potato, squash, and citrus fruits
- Red, blue, and purple berries of all kinds
- Green and white cruciferous vegetables like broccoli, cabbage, and cauliflower
- Red foods like tomatoes, red peppers, and watermelon
- Brown, red, tan, yellow, white, and green beans, lentils, and dried peas

Wholesome Habits

Cruciferous vegetables are named after the Latin word for *cross* since they bear cross-shaped flowers. Most are in the cabbage family and its relatives like broccoli and cauliflower, but they also include kale, mustard greens, collards, turnips, and rutabagas. Research shows these foods are excellent cancer-fighters and significantly inhibit growth of all types of tumors.

Processed Uncovered

Clean foods are foods without any man-made ingredients or unnecessary food additives. Food additives may be natural or artificial. Natural food additives include things like sugar, salt, corn syrup, pepper, and baking soda. Most natural food additives are generally recognized as safe and so are not subject to food safety regulation. Artificial or man-made additives, like artificial colors, flavors, and sweeteners are monitored and include a wide range of substances. To date, the FDA has approved more than 300 synthetic food additives for use in foods.

Spotting highly processed foods isn't as simple as you might think, particularly since some food additives—like salt and pepper—are natural. So, how do you know if an ingredient is necessary or not? If you're looking at a label and are unsure whether or not to buy a food, ask yourself the following questions:

- Are the ingredients natural or artificial?
- Are all these ingredients really necessary?
- Can I buy this product without these food additives and ingredients?

Certainly not all food additives are bad—think of rennet needed to make cheese, live active cultures added to yogurt, and the vitamins and minerals that enrich milk and cereal. But do we really need bread that will last two weeks on the shelf?

Ultimately, you'll determine what kinds of processed foods to include in your diet based on the cost of the foods, your lifestyle, and level of commitment to a clean eating diet.

Can the Carbs

Mother Nature provides a bounty of complex carbohydrates in fruits, vegetables, whole grains, and legumes. In the body, these carbs give us the energy that fuels our muscles and feeds our brain. So why get rid of them? You don't get rid of all of them—just the bad ones. Complex carbohydrates are considered "good carbs" because they are nutrient dense and often found in the company of fiber, vitamins, and minerals. They're essential for good health. Studies show they lower the risk of chronic illness, keep you regular, and are digested slowly, so energy is released at a steady pace, ensuring you can perform your best throughout the day. Complex carbohydrates are the foundation of the clean eating diet.

"Bad" carbohydrates are highly refined and processed, making them automatically off-limits when eating clean. They are mostly found in packaged or processed foods—strike two against them—and although they are a concentrated source of calories, they contribute very little nutritionally to your daily diet, making them bad news for people watching their weight. Strike three—you're out. The most common refined carbohydrates are white flour, white sugar, and white rice.

White Out Your Diet

Let's take a closer look at white flour. During processing, manufacturers remove the nutrient dense bran and germ of the wheat kernel, leaving only the starchy part and some protein. This kernel is then finely ground and sometimes bleached, yielding the white fluffy stuff we know so well. The same thing happens to white rice, minus the grinding process. The problem is the bran and germ contain hard-to-replace vitamins and minerals. Plus, the more processed the carbohydrate, the easier it is to digest and to absorb, causing fluctuations in blood sugar levels. Because refined carbs digest more quickly than complex carbs, you are more likely to eat large quantities of refined carbs, resulting in weight gain. Taking the white out of your diet not only slims you down, but introduces your taste buds to a whole new world of unusual tastes and textures.

Since whole grain flours are not as all-purpose as white flour, varying in protein, gluten (a type of protein that gives bread its stretch), and starch content, you'll need to experiment with different types and blends, especially when baking. Popular picks are as follows:

- **100 percent whole wheat flour,** made from hard red wheat, is the workhorse of the whole grain flours and can be used in most baked goods.

- **Whole wheat pastry flour** is a finer ground flour that produces a lighter, cakey texture and tender crumb.

- **Whole wheat white flour,** made from hard white wheat rather than red wheat, is lighter in color and softer in texture, making it a bit easier to bake with.

Other whole grain flours include oat, barley, spelt (with a light texture, this blends well with wheat and is one of my favorites), flaxseed meal, whole cornmeal, rye, buckwheat, and brown rice flour.

In addition to whole grain flours, clean eaters often take advantage of whole grains and brown rice. Whole grains that are making their way (or have already) into mainstream markets are rolled oats, cracked wheat, wheat berries, bulgur, barley, faro, spelt, amaranth, quinoa, millet, and buckwheat groats (kasha). Brown rice in all its variations—short, long, medium, basmati, even Japanese sushi—is now widely available as well.

> **Clean Cuts**
>
> Because whole grains and flours contain both the fibrous bran part and the oily germ part, they can turn rancid quickly, particularly if you live in a warm climate. To keep them fresh, seal them tightly and store in the refrigerator or freezer as soon as you bring them home.

Sugar Alternatives

Simple carbohydrates in the form of sugars satisfy a sweet tooth and provide a burst of energy. White table sugar is essentially pure sucrose, stripped of all its vitamins and minerals during processing. High-fructose corn syrup and pure fructose, although natural, are also highly refined. Fortunately for clean eaters, there are plenty of other natural unrefined sweeteners to take their place, including the following:

- **Agave nectar or syrup.** A popular sweetener from the Mexican agave cactus (which also gives us tequila), agave is 25 to 40 percent sweeter than table sugar. It ranges in color from light to dark amber and doesn't give you the spike in glucose other sweeteners do.

◆ **Date sugar.** With 60 percent sugar, dates are one of the sweetest fruits on Earth. Date sugar is simply dried dates ground into a powder—nothing more natural than that.

◆ **Honey.** Although only slightly sweeter than table sugar and with similar calories, honey is most prized for its rich, aromatic flavor. It is easy to digest and is believed to have antibacterial properties.

◆ **Maple syrup.** Made from the sap of maple trees, maple syrup is rich in minerals like manganese and zinc and contains fewer calories than honey.

◆ **Dehydrated (not evaporated) sugar cane juice.** This is cane sugar that has been cut, crushed, heated with water, and then dehydrated. It naturally contains molasses, some B vitamins, and minerals like calcium, potassium, and iron. Since the grainy crystals have less sucrose (and fewer calories) than table sugar, it tastes less sweet. The most common and widely used brand is Sucanat.

◆ **Stevia.** Stevia comes from the leaf of a plant native to Paraguay and has a slight licorice-like taste. It is 300 times sweeter than table sugar with zero-calories. For years it was only available as a dietary supplement, but recently it was approved by the FDA as a tabletop sweetener and for use in beverages. You can also cook with it, in small amounts.

Protein Power

How much protein do we really need? Recommended Dietary Allowances for protein are at ⅓ gram per pound of body weight—or 45 to 55 grams—of protein daily for average normal weight men and women. Physically active people, athletes, and older adults may need more—some experts say as much as twice that amount depending on how active you are. Even so, average American protein intakes can easily reach 95 grams per day. So, getting enough protein isn't a problem. More important is the quality of the protein and how you eat it.

Wholesome Habits

The Institute of Medicine says we should get at least 10 percent and no more than 35 percent of our total daily calories from protein. So the more calories you consume the more protein you'll need. One ounce of meat or ½ cup of legumes delivers 7 grams of protein.

Maximizing Your Potential

Eating clean means eating some sort of protein at every meal. To maximize its value, you should pair protein with carbohydrates and fats. The combination ensures you feel satisfied and energy levels stay on an even keel.

Among its many functions, protein builds strong bones and muscles. It's responsible for growth maintenance and repair. To get the most from your meals you have to pay attention to protein quality. Lean meat, fish, and chicken are nutrient dense and have everything you need, including all the *essential amino acids*, in one neat little package. Plus you don't need much of these foods to pack in enough protein.

> **Clean Cuts**
>
> Proteins are composed of **amino acids.** There are 20 amino acids altogether. Essential amino acids are the 9 amino acids you can only get through diet. The body can make the remaining nonessential amino acids, assuming the diet is adequate in essential amino acids.

High-Quality Options

The key to making good protein choices is watching your fat and calories. Since animal proteins tend to be high in fat and calories, this takes some vigilance. Certain foods—like lean beef and pork tenderloin, turkey and chicken breast—are naturally clean eating staples. Here are a few others we've found:

◆ **Eggs** are an excellent source of high-quality protein. Unfortunately, they're also high in fat. Although most of the protein is in the white, you'll be missing valuable nutrients if you consistently toss out the yolk, so instead of worrying about calories simply use one or two egg whites for every egg yolk and you can't go wrong.

> **Wholesome Habits**
>
> Greek yogurt is thicker and creamier than regular yogurt and has a lot less tang. It's also higher in protein than regular yogurt. Used as an all-purpose spread, dip, and sauce, it's indispensable in the clean kitchen.

◆ **Low-fat dairy** like reduced fat or nonfat milk, low-fat sour cream, cottage cheese, cheese, and cream cheese is also essential. With almost half the sodium of milk, less than one quarter the amount of sugar, and fewer calories, unsweetened soymilk has become a standard in my household. Greek yogurt—either nonfat or low-fat—is another favorite.

- **Shellfish** such as shrimp, clams, and mussels are all good bets and leaner and lower in calories than most fin fish.

- **Lean ground beef** (93 or 95 percent lean) is another good choice. When buying ground turkey be sure and check the label as some brands include fat and skin.

Protein Powders and Supplements

Many active people who follow a clean lifestyle load up on protein with protein powders and supplements. Unfortunately, they're probably just wasting their money. Most Americans, even those who are physically active, can easily meet their protein needs through a healthy diet.

Too much protein not only increases your likelihood of gaining weight (by increasing calories), but it can also stress your kidneys and increase water and calcium losses. If you still feel the need to use protein powders and supplements they can be added to many of the drink and smoothie recipes in Chapters 6 and 12.

Avoid the Fear Factor: Fat

There are plenty of reasons to avoid eating too much fat. First of all, consuming too much fat makes you fat. Fat also increases your risk for chronic illness, and consuming too many fatty foods leaves little room for more nutritious foods. The worst fat offenders are saturated fats and trans fats.

Saturated fats are found in the visible white fat and fatty streaks in rich cuts of red meat. In chicken it's found primarily in the skin and dark meat. Plants aren't immune to saturated fat, either. Coconut oil, palm oil, palm kernel oil, and cocoa butter are loaded with saturated fat. Clean eaters minimize their intake of these fats.

Trans fats are man-made fats found in fried foods, store-bought cookies, cakes, icings, and other processed foods. They should be completely eliminated from your diet because they raise blood cholesterol levels. Fortunately, trans fats have recently been banned in many restaurants and foodservice establishments in cities across the country, including New York City. Most food manufacturers have also stopped using them.

Get Mono

Despite fat's negative reputation, cutting out all fats is a bad idea. Some fat is vital for good health. And a diet without fat would be bland and boring. That's where mono-unsaturated fats come into play. Research shows monounsaturated fats do not promote heart disease, stroke, cancer, and various other conditions; and they may even protect you against them. Olive oil is the most famous source of these celebrity fats, but there are plenty of other sources as well—avocadoes, canola oil, nuts (all kinds), and nut butters. Seeds and seed oils are also abundant in monounsaturated fat.

But just because a fat is good for you doesn't mean you can eat as much of it as you want. Most clean eating recipes use one or two teaspoons of olive oil at the most, and nuts and avocados, although an important part of a clean eating diet, should be used sparingly.

Forget Frying

Few people realize how much oil they use during the actual cooking process. I know I didn't. In order to eat clean you may need to revamp your cooking style.

Pan-frying and deep fat frying are the worst cooking methods because they are high in fat and calories. Neither of these methods are acceptable on the clean eating plan. Consider that a battered and fried $1/2$ chicken breast weighs in at 364 calories and 18 grams of fat, whereas the same baked or grilled skinless chicken breast has only 142 calories and 3 grams of fat. What a difference! Even vegetables are not worth eating when dripping with fat.

Sautéeing and stir-frying, although better cooking methods, can be just as unhealthy if you pour on the oil. The key is to keep the fats in check by using only small amounts of oil.

Although grilling might seem like an ideal clean eating cooking technique because it doesn't require the use of any oils, it, too, has its pitfalls. Unfortunately, high temperatures produce cancer-causing compounds called heterocyclic amines (HA) in red meat and chicken. HA's are notoriously concentrated in the black grill marks you often see in foods served at restaurants. The solution—lower the heat. Keep the grill at low to moderate temperatures and don't let any flames shoot up.

Wholesome Habits _____

Worried about carcinogens in your grilled meat? Marinate them first. In a recent Portuguese study, marinating beef for up to six hours in red wine or beer before cooking reduced heterocyclic amines (HA's) by 40 percent and 88 percent respectively. Marinating meat in herb blends containing rosemary or oregano also decreased HA formation.

Mini Me

The typical clean diet features three small main meals and two to three substantial snacks every day. Eating this way prevents you from overeating, skipping meals, and feeling fatigued or jittery from unstable blood sugar levels. It also helps you lose weight. Several studies show people who eat small frequent meals accumulate less fat than those who eat the same number of calories in fewer larger meals.

By substantial snacks, we mean 100 to 200 calories in each snack. All snacks, as well as meals, should include balanced portions of protein, fat, and carbohydrates. One of my favorite snacks is a hard-boiled egg with some crackers; another is a sliced banana topped with almond butter sprinkled with a bit of dark chocolate, all rolled in a whole wheat flour tortilla (see recipe in Chapter 9).

Main meals should generally range from 200 to 400 calories. This is considerably smaller than most Americans are used to eating but you won't miss out with dishes like Beef Tenderloin with Asparagus and Toasted Barley (see recipe in Chapter 18). A 1-cup serving of the beef-vegetable mixture served over a 1-cup serving of barley has only 337 calories. Since you eat so frequently, hunger isn't a big deal. The biggest issue is getting used to your new lifestyle of eating often and in small portions.

Here are a few tips that can make the transition easier:

◆ Portion out everything, especially at first, so you know what a proper serving size is.

◆ Carry a cooler with snacks in the car.

◆ Keep a stash of clean food at the office.

◆ Buy smaller dinner plates, bowls, and cups, so your plate will still look full even though you're eating less.

◆ Be prepared; plan all snacks, lunches, and dinners ahead of time.

Wet Your Whistle with Water

Water makes up about 60 percent of the human body, and it is involved in every system in the body. It regulates body temperature, cushions and protects vital organs, transports nutrients, and eliminates waste.

So how much water should you drink? For years health organizations recommended 8 (8-ounce) glasses of water a day *in addition* to your other beverages, but these guidelines have lightened up. While drinking 8 glasses of water is still a good idea, if you don't meet that goal don't beat yourself up. The 2006 Healthy Beverage Guidelines say drinking $2^{1}/_{2}$ to 6 (8-ounce glasses) of water a day plus other beverages is perfectly acceptable. Here's what you need to do to keep your body clean and healthy:

Dirty Secrets

Muscle is about 75 percent water, while only about 10 percent of fat cells are composed of water.

Drink when you're thirsty. Thirst and hunger are two separate mechanisms; unfortunately, many people mistake thirst for hunger, which leads to piling on unnecessary calories.

Sip rather than gulp. Keep a glass of water nearby to sip throughout the day.

Drink a glass before meals. Many people drink a glass of water before dinner to fill themselves up, so they eat less. If this works for you, go for it.

Make water your first choice. Americans consume 21 percent of their daily calories from beverages. Few people are aware of all the "liquid calories" they drink. Sugar-sweetened sodas with high-fructose corn syrup or other refined sugars are not included on a clean diet. Water is your best bet. If you do want something else, choose natural fruit juices. To cut the sugars dilute these drinks by 50 percent with water, sparkling water, or seltzer.

Know when to drink more. If you are physically active, sweat a lot, live in a hot climate, or are sick, you need more water. To prevent dehydration when you exercise, drink before, during, and after workouts. An extra $1^{1}/_{2}$ to $2^{1}/_{2}$ cups is all you need for short exercise bouts of an hour or so.

Eat foods with high water content. Lettuce, broccoli, watermelon, and yogurt contain more than 85 percent water. Foods high in water volume—like broth-based soups, fruits, vegetables, and oatmeal—boost your fullness factor so you eat less.

Dirty Secrets _____

Before you go out for a night on the town, consider that 1 (5-ounce) glass of wine, red or white, supplies 120 empty calories. Too much alcohol can also affect your performance in the gym and disrupt sleep. Sports drinks and sweetened caffeinated drinks are also usually loaded with calories. Limiting caffeine drinks like coffee is also a good idea, particularly if you are sensitive to its effects.

The best clean drink choices:

◆ Water

◆ Unsweetened tea

◆ 100 percent pure fruit juice (drink sparingly)

◆ Low-fat or skim milk and unsweetened low-fat soymilk

Move It!

The eating clean lifestyle is an active lifestyle that involves exercising 5 or 6 times a week, 30 to 60 minutes a day. In addition to making you look great and feel fabulous, working out regularly has plenty of other benefits. First, regular exercise slims you down by decreasing fat and building muscle. Having more muscle raises your metabolism, so that you burn more energy even at rest, making it easier to keep the weight off. Exercise also acts like a natural appetite suppressant, curbing cravings and hunger pangs.

Physically, working out strengthens your heart and lungs, builds strong bones, jump-starts your immune system, and produces glowing skin, not to mention reducing your risk for chronic illnesses. Since muscle weighs more than fat (because it contains more water) it's also possible to lose inches without budging the scale.

Mentally, exercise improves mood, counters depression, and makes you feel good. Clean eaters who also regularly exercise report better sleep, clearer mental focus, and less stress.

Vary Your Routine

The key to keeping fit is not getting bored with your routine. Shake up the following components in your weekly workouts to maximize your health.

Aerobic activity. This cardiovascular exercise is good for the heart and includes running, biking, and brisk walking. Since most aerobic exercises are weight bearing they're also good for preventing bone loss. A good mix is to alternate between vigorous and moderate intensity workouts.

Muscle strengthening. Strength training and toning is essential for keeping you strong and preventing muscle loss, which naturally occurs as we age. If you're a woman, don't worry about becoming too muscular; most women don't have the genes to bulk up.

Core training. This tightens the abs, improves balance, and protects the back. Core conditioning develops functional fitness, which is required for daily routine activities.

Flexibility. Flexibility helps decrease the risk of injuries, and unfortunately we become less flexible as we age. The best time to stretch is after your workout when you are warmed up.

Fitting It In

If you make exercise a priority in your life, it will become habit, and habits are hard to break.

Wholesome Habits _____

For each pound of muscle you add to your body, you will burn an additional 35 to 50 calories per day.

The best way to get into the habit of exercising is to do it the same time every day. This also helps your body better adjust to the new routine. When you work out depends on your lifestyle. But the most important thing is that you do it every day.

The Least You Need to Know

◆ Clean eating is based on eating natural, whole, unprocessed foods that are high in protein and low in fat and sugar.

◆ Refined carbohydrates like white sugar and white flour lack nutrients and supply empty calories; they should be minimized or eliminated altogether from your diet.

- Eating 5 or 6 small balanced meals throughout the day will keep your energy level high and prevent you from overeating.

- Make water your drink of choice. Also make it a point to choose foods and meals with high water content.

- Regular exercise is an essential part of the clean eating lifestyle and offers a wealth of benefits.

3

Cleaning Up Your Act

In This Chapter

- ◆ Deciphering food labels
- ◆ Cleaning up your kitchen
- ◆ Time- and money-saving planning tips
- ◆ Smart shopping hints
- ◆ Eating clean while eating out

Now that you know the basic principles of a clean eating lifestyle, it's time to start making changes. Like all change, eating clean may seem awkward at first, but it will get easier quickly, and the payoffs of losing unwanted pounds and having good health, vitality, and energy will make it all worthwhile. When I first started preparing clean meals for my family, they often complained about the extra time and effort it took. But after only a week of clean eating we all felt and looked better, and I became more efficient in the kitchen. Now I wouldn't dream of going back to eating meals from boxes and packages.

Clean eating starts at home, and I found the best way to start is to go cold turkey. This chapter shows you how to purge the pantry, fridge, and freezer of processed foods, plan out your meals, and be a smart food shopper. The biggest reason people eat processed food is not taste or even price, but convenience. That's why not having any clean food prepared or planned is the kiss of death. It's almost impossible not to reach for that high-fat, high-calorie, salty frozen dinner when your stomach is growling and there's nothing else to eat.

Although restaurants are notorious for rich sauces and calorie-laden dishes, it is possible to stay clean while dining out as long as you plan ahead and choose carefully. This chapter gives you tips for navigating the menu and enjoying eating out clean.

Learning Label Lingo

It's easy to choose clean food in the produce aisle—almost everything there is a good choice—but for almost every other type of food you have to read food labels. The label tells you if the product contains any unwanted ingredients and the amounts of fat, sodium, sugar, and calories in the product. Most processed foods are packed with unnecessary calories, which is why cutting them out helps you automatically slim down.

You don't need a food science degree to decipher food labels, but you do need to learn the lingo. Every food label has two parts: the nutrition facts panel and the ingredient list.

The Nutrition Facts Panel

The nutrition facts panel gives you a quick nutritional snapshot of the food. It contains amounts for calories, fat calories, total fat, saturated fat, trans fats, cholesterol, sodium, total carbohydrates, dietary fiber, sugars, and protein. To give you an idea of how these numbers fit into your diet, the label also lists the percent of recommended daily values provided by the food. These daily values are based on a 2,000 calorie diet with 30 percent of calories coming from fat, with 10 percent of those fat calories from saturated fat, 60 percent calories from carbohydrates, and 10 percent calories from protein. Fiber is set at 25 grams per day, and sodium at 2,400 milligrams per day.

As noted in Chapter 2, you want to purchase foods that are high in fiber and low in fats, sugars, and sodium, with low calories. Since you'll be eating 5 or 6 times a day, you won't go hungry but you'll still lose weight.

Clean foods are not based on nutritional label daily values. They are lower in fat, calories, sugar, cholesterol, and sodium and higher in protein. When you're reading labels you want to look at specific gram amounts rather than percentages. Each of the recipes in this book strive for …

♦ 10 grams of total fat or less and no more than 15 grams.

♦ 8 to 10 grams of sugar or less for main meals and sides and no more than 20 grams for snacks, desserts, and drinks.

♦ 100 mg cholesterol or less.

♦ 500 to 550 mg sodium or less.

If you keep these numbers in line, all the rest of the nutrients for calories, carbo-hydrates, and protein fall in line.

> **Wholesome Habits** _____
>
> Percent daily values can also tell you whether a food contributes a little or a lot of a certain nutrient like calcium, iron, or fiber. If the food has 20 percent or more of the recommended daily value it can be labeled as a "high" or an "excellent" source, 10 to 19 percent is considered a "good" source, and 5 percent or less is a low source.

The Ingredient List

Reading ingredient lists is essential to eating clean. By law, all packaged food sold in retail stores must list all the foods contained in that product. However, if an ingredient falls under 0.5 grams per serving the manufacturer can list it as being "0" on the nutrition facts panel.

Reading the ingredient lists lets you know if there are any excess sugars and salts or unnecessary chemical additives, like preservatives, emulsifiers, stabilizers, or artificial colors and flavors in the food. Here's a brief explanation of each of these substances:

♦ **Preservatives** prevent foods from spoiling by protecting fats from going rancid and vegetables and fruits from turning brown. They also stop the growth of mold, bacteria, and yeast.

♦ **Emulsifiers** keep water and oil in foods from separating.

♦ **Stabilizers** and **thickeners** maintain a smooth texture and uniform color and flavor in food.

♦ **Colors and flavors** enhance the appearance and taste of the food. Artificial colors are man-made food dyes such as Yellow #5. Natural colors come from foods and include beetroot powder, caramel color (made from heating sugar until it turns brown), and beta-carotene; these are better choices than artificial colors. Both natural and artificial flavors are isolated chemical compounds created in a lab by chemists or "flavorists."

A clean eating lifestyle seeks to minimize all of these components in food.

Dirty Secrets

Beware: the nutrition facts panel may list the amount of trans fat as 0, but the food could still include up to 0.5 grams of partially hydrogenated or hydrogenated oils in their lineup.

A product's ingredients are listed in descending order by weight. Thus, the first ingredient is always what the food contains the most of.

When it comes to ingredients, the shorter the list, the better. Not only are short lists of 5 to 10 ingredients less likely to have a lot of additives, they're also more likely to contain recognizable ingredients like olive oil, tomatoes, and red peppers, that you can find in your kitchen, rather than in a laboratory.

As a general rule, try not to buy foods with ingredients you can't pronounce. In particular, avoid foods with the following ingredients, as this means they are highly processed and may have some safety issues:

Butylated Hydroxyanisole (BHA) and Butylated Hydroxytoluene (BHT)   Both BHA and BHT keep fats from going rancid. They have been linked to cancer in animal studies. Safer, more natural substitutes are available on the market.

High-fructose corn syrup   A highly processed and refined sugar made from fructose and glucose; it is prevalent in our food supply and increases our risk of obesity.

Potassium bromate   A dough conditioner that has been linked to cancer in animal studies.

Sodium/potassium benzoate   A preservative used in soft drinks and fruit drinks. When combined with vitamin C it may form benzene, a known carcinogen. Many manufacturers have eliminated this risk, but some have not.

Propyl gallate   A preservative, usually combined with BHT and BHA, which may increase risk of cancer.

Sodium nitrate/nitrites   Preservatives found in cured meats that give them their characteristic red color. Nitrites have been shown to cause cancer in lab animals. Nitrates are converted to nitrites in the body.

Artificial colors and flavors (natural and artificial) and numbered dyes such as red 40, yellow 5, or blue 2   Not only are these man-made substances highly processed and largely unnecessary, many (especially the dyes) are thought to be cancer-causing.

Also pass on artificial sweeteners such as aspartame, sucralose, saccharin, acesulfame-K; the flavor enhancer monosodium glutamate (MSG); and hydrogenated and partially hydrogenated fats. The safety of artificial sweeteners has been a controversial issue for decades. Furthermore, artificial sweeteners are not part of a healthy clean diet. Aside from adding extra salt to the diet, MSG can cause migraines, nausea, and fatigue in sensitive individuals. Hydrogenated fats increase the risk of heart disease.

Beware of other added sugars or sweeteners, which can appear in many disguises, sometimes showing up several times on one ingredient list. All of these terms are simply another way of saying sugar:

Corn syrup	Dextrin
High-fructose corn syrup	Maltodextrin
Molasses	Brown sugar
Honey	Brown rice syrup
Dextrose	Sorghum syrup
Evaporated cane juice	Beet sugar
Agave nectar	Cane sugar
Maple syrup	Raw sugar
Sucrose	Invert sugar
Fructose	Turbinado sugar

If you buy any packaged foods, choose minimally processed products with little or no synthetic ingredients and few preservatives, stabilizers, emulsifiers, and colors.

If they have these ingredients, make sure they are natural and safe, like carrageenan (made from seaweed or algae), guar gum, citric acid (from citrus fruits), ascorbic acid (vitamin C), and beta-carotene (for color). For a comprehensive list of food additives check out www.cspinet.org/reports/chemcuisine.htm.

Cleaning House

Filling your pantry with clean, wholesome foods is the first step in a sustainable clean eating lifestyle. While some energetic people jump right in and start eating clean immediately, others make a more gradual transition, slowly switching out processed foods for more whole fruits and vegetables and moving from white flour to whole grains in small steps.

For those who rely on processed foods for most of their meals, I recommend a slow transition. This gives your taste buds time to adjust to less salt and sugar, gives you more time to adapt to the clean eating lifestyle, and enables you to reorganize your pantry bit by bit, which may be more cost effective if you've stockpiled frozen dinners and box mixes.

Either way, when it comes to eating healthy and low-fat, the best strategy is "out-of-sight, out-of-mind." By eliminating all processed foods from your kitchen you remove temptation and make room for more wholesome, natural foods.

What should you do with all the processed foods you no longer want? You can donate them (if unopened) to a food pantry, give them away to someone you know, throw them out, or use them up gradually. Since most processed foods are made to last a long time, keeping them is usually not a problem. If you do decide to hold on to them, put them on a separate shelf in the farthest part of the fridge or freezer or in a box far back in your cupboards. Eventually you will lose your taste for them altogether.

Pantry Purge

Now let's take a look at some of the most common processed foods and where they hide.

Foods in a box. These include meals like macaroni and cheese, skillet dinners, and soup mixes; packaged side dishes like prepared rices, pastas and noodles, and scalloped or mashed potatoes; certain crackers; sugary cereals; sweets like boxed cakes, cookies, puddings, custards, and jellos; prepared breadcrumbs; seasoning packages like taco mix, dry sauce mixes, and anything labeled "instant."

Store-bought condiments and sauces. Any food listing high-fructose corn syrup as the first, second, or third ingredient is out. This means ketchup, most barbecue sauces, jams, jellies, and many Asian sauces like duck sauce, hoisin, and stir-fry sauce. High-fat and high-sodium products like full-fat mayonnaise and regular soy sauce are also off-limits.

Canned meals like soups, stews, and chili. These products are generally loaded with salt, sugar, fat, artificial preservatives, and highly processed ingredients like modified food starch, corn syrup solids, and maltodextrin. However, low sodium chicken, vegetable, or beef broth are okay to use sparingly since they are minimally processed and contain few ingredients. Low sodium canned beans and tomato products are also okay in a pinch, as are canned evaporated skim milk, and pumpkin and fruits that are packed in their own juice without added sugar. But remember, the majority of your fruits and vegetables should be bought fresh, so cans should only be used as backup. If you do keep some on hand, be sure and read the ingredient label first—even canned vegetables like peas and corn can have sugar added.

Refined white flour and white sugar. For many people the hardest part of going clean is eliminating refined white flour and white sugar. This means getting rid of all-purpose white flour, granulated white sugar, regular pasta, white bread, white crackers, and white rice, and replacing them with whole grain alternatives.

Clean Cuts _____
If you have an open bag of white flour and don't want to throw it out, you can mix it with whole wheat flour in recipes. Typically, whole wheat flour can be substituted for 50 percent of white flour in recipes without drastically altering taste and texture.

Refrigerator Raid

Whole milk, eggs, butter, sour cream, cheese, and cream cheese are high in fat and saturated fat. Some people can eliminate them from their diet completely without any bother, others can't imagine going without. For the latter group, there are two choices: replacing them with low-fat products and limiting portion sizes. In this book I've included recipes using both those alternatives, so don't be surprised to see a dab of butter or a whole egg or two in a recipe.

Eliminate fat-free foods, too. Most fat-free foods replace the fat with sugars, modified starch, and other unnatural ingredients. Low-fat versions are better choices because they are less processed, with the exception of skim milk and those products made with skim milk like 0 percent fat yogurt and certain soft cheeses.

Toss anything containing high-fructose corn syrup, artificial sweeteners, or high levels of sugar. Other high sugar items include fruit yogurt, puddings, and chocolate and flavored milk or yogurt-based drinks.

Not only are precooked, prepared meats like bacon, bologna, hot dogs, and ham high in fat and calories, they're also full of salt, nitrites, and nitrates. High intakes of nitrites and nitrates have been linked to an increased risk of cancer.

Freezer Fall Out

Store-bought frozen dinners, including frozen pizzas, are heavily processed and often run high in sodium, calories, and fat. They also lack fiber. To make up for the loss of these easy meals, you'll be making your own frozen dinners, which are much healthier and just as convenient.

Avoid all prepared frozen vegetables that are lightly seasoned; doused in butter, cheese, or cream sauces; or breaded and fried. The same holds true for bread, noodle, potato, or rice dishes.

Frozen snacks are a no-no. Ditch the bagel bites, pizza, mozzarella sticks, tacos, potato skins, chicken wings, burritos, mini eggrolls, and spinach dips. Not only are they unclean, they rack up calories fast. And as you probably guessed, frozen desserts go, too. This covers premium novelty desserts, toppings, and most ice creams.

So What *Can* You Eat?

Plenty! Eating clean emphasizes fresh, natural foods that are minimally processed if at all. Fresh fruits, vegetables, meat, fish, and poultry are the mainstays of the diet, along with whole grains and dried beans. But that doesn't mean the diet is sugar-free, fat-free, or lacks flavor. Natural unrefined sweeteners, nut butters, and monounsaturated oils are also part of the diet. The key is balancing these ingredients in your meals. Once you get the hang of it, you'll find that eating clean will actually expand your culinary horizons and offer you a wider variety of better-tasting food choices.

Managing Your Time

There's no question that when you commit to a clean eating lifestyle you'll be spending more time in the kitchen preparing meals. In return you will have healthy, high-quality, low-fat meals that will make you feel fit and energized. This doesn't mean you will be spending hours in the kitchen every night. In fact, Chapter 16 is devoted to making meals in 30 minutes or less. But eating well does require more planning than simply grabbing a microwaveable dinner or stopping at your local fast-food restaurant.

Remember, too, cooking is a skill, and like any skill, the more you do it the more accomplished you will become. So, go ahead and try the recipes in this book. Don't be afraid to tackle some of the longer, more complicated options when you have the time. Since they make big batches and lend themselves to freezing, you will save time in the long run. Eventually you'll be whipping up low-calorie flavorful meals in a flash.

Wholesome Habits

In 1965, a married woman who didn't work spent more than two hours per day cooking and cleaning up from meals. By 1995, the same tasks took less than half that time. Today, most people expect a meal to be prepared in 15 to 20 minutes and to use fewer than 6 ingredients. But saving time doesn't mean saving calories; in fact, the opposite may be true. Over the last 40 years, average daily calorie consumption has risen by 500 calories and obesity rates have doubled.

Be Well-Equipped

Having the right kitchen tools is essential for preparing clean food and saving time. Don't bother buying any fancy kitchen gadgets or gizmos—you don't need them. Just start with the basics for now, and add to your kitchen slowly as you get more proficient. Here is a list of what you should have:

- A high-quality, heavy-duty 8-inch chef's knife with a stainless steel blade.

- A good 3-inch paring knife.

- A knife sharpener.

- Two sturdy plastic cutting boards. Reserve one for cutting raw meat, fish, or poultry and the other for everything else. Color-coded boards are great for this.

- A good set of nonstick pots and pans made of hard-anodized aluminum.

Wholesome Habits

Having sharp knives makes a huge difference when it comes to preparing clean meals. It will make slicing, chopping and dicing faster, easier and neater—instead of pushing your knife through the food you merely guide it. If you're cooking clean regularly, a quality knife should last between six months to a year before it needs sharpening.

◆ A well-seasoned cast-iron pan. Stainless steel is also a good conductor of heat, but requires the use of fat, as the food tends to stick without it.

◆ A food scale and a set of measuring spoons and cups

◆ A pizza/baking stone. Baking stones do not require any oil to prevent foods from sticking and so help clean eaters reduce the amount of fat in their diets.

◆ A set of plastic storage containers for the freezer and refrigerator. Be sure to have plenty of small pieces for bringing lunch and snacks to work.

Kitchen Shortcuts

To make the most of your time in the kitchen, it helps to know some cooking tips and techniques. When preparing a meal from a recipe, always read the recipe first, before you start cooking. Then make sure you have all the ingredients, proper utensils, and cookware ready and prepped.

> **Wholesome Habits**
>
> In the culinary world, chefs are trained in *mise en place,* a French culinary phrase that literally means "to put in place." This refers to having all the ingredients and tools you need for a dish ready before you start. Vegetables, meats, seasonings, and sauces are all prepped and set aside. Good mise en place is one of the reasons why restaurant chefs are able to serve so many meals in one night.

Other ways to save on time are to get friendly with your freezer. Keep a stash of frozen fruits and vegetables, which you can defrost quickly or cook directly from their frozen state. Ideally, you've frozen these foods yourself from their fresh state, during peak season when they are at their ripest and most plentiful.

Most vegetables must be blanched or roasted first, then portioned and frozen. Fruits like blueberries and blackberries can be wrapped and frozen straight from the store or garden. If you want to freeze individual pieces, such as strawberries or cauliflower, just put the pieces on a baking pan and freeze for about 1 hour; once frozen, you can take them off the baking pan and place them in an airtight freezer bag. Always date and label each product.

Store-bought frozen fruits and vegetables are good choices when fresh are not available. Just make sure there are no extra ingredients added in such as sugar or salt.

Avoid vegetables in butter sauces and with added flavoring. Because fruits and vegetables are flash frozen—usually hours after being picked—they maintain most of their nutritional value.

Washed and bagged lettuce, spinach, and other greens are welcome shortcuts, too. Although physically processed, these foods don't have any additives or preservatives. They do have a much shorter shelf life than unwashed and uncut produce. For this reason you usually need to use them within a few days.

> **Clean Cuts**
> Draining and rinsing canned beans can reduce the sodium content by 40 percent. This drops a ½ cup serving of chickpeas from 360 mg of sodium to only 216 mg.

Packaged produce usually has a best-used-by-date, which signifies peak quality. Sometimes it's okay to use after the date, but taste and texture may be altered. The shelf life of fresh produce, not bagged, can range from 2 to 7 days to 1 month from purchase depending on the produce. Keep in mind that when it comes to nutritional quality, the sooner you eat it the better. For more information about handling and storing seasonal foods visit the FAQ section at www.farmernet.com.

Plan Ahead

Of all the clean eating lifestyle changes, planning your meals in advance is the most important to ensuring success. Some of the best intentions have gone down the drain simply because of lack of planning. Master the art of menu planning and you have the keys to success right in your hand. Here's what you need to know:

Build a well-stocked pantry, fridge, and freezer. This ensures stocks, soups, sauces, beans, and grains are at the ready when you need them. Portion them in reasonable containers. Cook up a big batch of brown rice, and you have instant rice, ready to be reheated, three days later. Check out Chapter 17 for make-ahead dinner ideas.

Bake ahead. Baked items like whole grain breads, muffins, and scones freeze beautifully. When divvied up in individual portions they are perfect for a quick grab-and-go breakfast or snack in the afternoon.

Plan all your meals. Make a menu for 5 to 7 days and include breakfast, lunch, dinner, and all your snacks. Then stick to it. You may switch around meals or snacks, but keep to the general pattern. Prepare at least one meal and one side dish that can do double duty and be revamped later in the week. See Appendix B for a sample menu plan.

You Gotta Shop Around

Since conventional grocery stores tend to stock a limited amount of produce and mostly highly processed foods, you'll need to shop around. You can still get plenty of basics at conventional grocery stores, especially since many now have specialty store brands which are all natural and tend to be lower in fat, sugar, and calories. But when it comes to buying unrefined sugars and sweeteners and a variety of whole grains, flours, and breads, natural food stores are your best option—either big chains like Whole Foods, Trader Joe's, and Harris Teeter or small independent grocers and co-operatives. If you don't have any natural food stores nearby, you can do most of your shopping online.

For produce, start at your local farmers' market. They may not have the biggest selection, but they do have the freshest and most seasonal fruits and vegetables. To find out where there's a farmers' market near you, visit www.localharvest.org.

Ethnic markets are another avenue to explore. Not only do they boast a variety of unusual and interesting foods—especially produce—but they can often light the spark of culinary creativity and introduce you to a world of exotic herbs and spices.

Before You Go

Before you head to the store, create a list of ingredients needed for the menu you wrote for the week. Then check the ingredients list against your pantry, fridge, and freezer supplies. Based on your inventory, create a shopping list.

Dirty Secrets

If you have children, it's best to leave them at home when grocery shopping. Most junk food marketers target children (there's a reason why sugary cereals are placed on the lower shelves, exactly eye level with little ones), and few parents with kids in tow can avoid being cajoled into buying some sort of sugar-laden food. So do yourself a favor and leave the kids home.

And, finally, keep in mind that a hungry shopper often buys more food than he or she needs. To prevent your stomach from making your purchasing decisions, keep some snacks such as nuts and dried fruit in your car.

At the Store

As a clean eater, you'll find almost everything you need around the perimeter of the store, where most fresh items are located. Skip over the deli section as this usually houses fatty, processed meats and cheeses. When considering processed foods from the interior of the store, pay close attention to the labels, and be sure to compare different brands. For instance, when shopping for apple butter a while back, the ingredient label on the first brand I picked up listed apples, high-fructose corn syrup, sugar, and water. Fortunately, another brand of apple butter had a much cleaner ingredient list: apples and apple cider.

Don't be fooled by labels that make health claims for their products. Many products touted as healthy are not as good as they look. Ignore the healthy name or claim and scan the nutrition facts panel and ingredients label before making any decisions.

Dirty Secrets

Beware of products labeled "reduced sugar," "less sugar," or "lite." More often than not, this means they contain artificial sweeteners. Don't assume less sugar equals less calories, either. Sometimes sugar-free or reduced sugar foods have as many or more calories than the original because of higher fat, starch, or protein content.

Eating Out, Eating Clean

Eating out can be challenging for clean eaters, but that's not to say you can't find a clean meal in a restaurant. Among the pitfalls you're likely to face are big portion sizes; rich sauces loaded with butter, oil, and cream; and too much salt. In addition, some restaurants do little cooking in-house, relying instead on preprepared convenience foods, which are high in salt, sugar, fat, and additives and preservatives. Here's what to do:

Go online. If the restaurant has a website, look at their menu online. Check out their philosophy (are they service oriented?) and look for healthier fare. Ideally, you want to have your menu choice picked out before you even walk through the door.

Think outside the box. Just because you're in a restaurant doesn't mean you have to order a meal. You can order two side vegetable dishes, a side salad or an appetizer, and a side dish as your entrée. Another option is to consider splitting a dinner or taking half of it home.

Talk to your waiter. Your waiter is your lifeline to the kitchen. Explain to him or her what you are looking for and what you want to avoid. Your server should be able to explain to you what's in every dish and how it is prepared. If he or she can't, ask them to check with the chef and let you know.

Clean Cuts

To read more about how to dine out healthy, check out *Eat Out, Eat Right: The Guide to Healthier Restaurant Eating* (third edition) by Hope Warshaw. Although not specifically targeted to eating clean, the book tells you how to find healthy, low-calorie nutritious meals at almost any type of restaurant.

Don't be afraid to make special requests. This is your most important tool for staying clean and eating low-fat, low-calorie meals. In fact, there are few restaurants where you won't ask for something changed. Order chicken without the sauce, whole grain bread instead of potato, or extra vegetables sans the butter, oil, and salt. Beware of red-light words like crispy, fried, buttery, garlic sauce, melted cheese, or herb sauce. Be firm and clear with your request and remember that most restaurants want to make their customers happy. Keep in mind that the more special requests you make, the more likely the kitchen will make a mistake. Try to find dishes on the menu that only need a few changes to accommodate your needs.

The Least You Need to Know

◆ Knowing how to decipher food labels is essential to eating clean.

◆ Highly processed foods have a long list of ingredients and are usually high in fat, calories, and sodium.

◆ Planning your menu a week in advance—and sticking with that menu—makes it easier to stick with a healthy diet.

◆ Eating clean when eating out requires extra vigilance and effort on your part, but it can be done.

Chapter 4

Super Secrets for Keeping Clean

In This Chapter

- ◆ Flavor boosters
- ◆ Why it pays to pack a snack
- ◆ Conquering temptation
- ◆ Cheats you can live with

With any kind of transition there are bound to be bumps in the road. This is particularly true if you're switching from a typical standard American diet and sedentary lifestyle to a clean eating, active life. Fortunately, you'll find plenty of ways to get past these roadblocks and follow a clean, healthy life.

In this chapter we confront some of the challenges committed clean eaters face, like adjusting to your new way of cooking; always having good, clean food within reach; and avoiding the temptations of junk food. Consider the suggestions we offer in this chapter as starting points to build on and personalize as you go. With each new eating experience, you gain valuable insight into how to deal with these and other issues. Who knows—with your new vitality and healthy glow, you may even inspire some converts.

Beat the Blahs

The biggest complaint of newbie clean eaters is that the food tastes bland. This is especially an issue for those who previously lived on a diet of frozen dinners and take-out. Clean food tastes bland at first because we have become accustomed to the high levels of sugar and salt in processed foods. The more we eat of these over-processed flavors, the more our taste buds become desensitized or resistant to their taste. Eventually, we crave more and more to fill this need. That's why food that tastes salty or overly sweet to one person doesn't taste that way at all to another. Getting your taste buds used to less salt and sugar takes weeks, sometimes even months, to achieve because they have to "re-learn" how to taste. In this case, it's best to go cold turkey, giving your taste buds time to "forget." Eventually junk foods may taste so salty or sweet you'll wonder how you ever ate them!

In addition, if you're new to cooking, you'll need to learn what kinds of seasonings—and in what quantities—to add to your dishes to enhance their flavor. Master the art of herbs and spices and your cooking will achieve entirely new levels of deliciousness.

Healthy Herbs and Spices

What, exactly, are herbs and spices? In the culinary world, herbs are the aromatic green leaves of a plant. Some of the most common herbs include parsley, dill, oregano, basil, cilantro, and thyme. Spices come from parts of plants, too—usually the bark, root, seeds, buds, or berries—and are usually whole, crushed, or ground. Some dehydrated and ground vegetables like garlic, onions, and chile peppers are also considered spices.

Herbs and spices can be the star of the meal or they can be subtle hints, rounding out the background flavors of a dish.

Dirty Secrets

Always read the label before buying prepared seasoning blends. Many have salt and sugar added to them.

Herbs and spices are ideal for boosting flavor when eating clean because they are completely natural, lack sodium and sugar, and have few calories. Fresh herbs are best, but if you're buying spices and dried herbs go for single ingredient products like dried parsley or paprika. Products labeled Italian spices or Creole spices are usually a mixture of different seasonings and can contain lots of artificial chemicals.

Perhaps the most appealing reason to up your intake of these flavoring agents is the beneficial antioxidants they bring to the table. Ounce for ounce, herbs and spices are nature's most concentrated source of antioxidants, beating out almost all fruits and vegetables. Oregano tops the list of herbs, with 20 times more antioxidant power than other herbs and 4 times more than blueberries. On the spice side, ground cloves rank number one, followed by cinnamon and then turmeric, the yellow colored spice that gives curry powder its distinctive flavor.

Seasoning your food with the proper herbs and spices can make the difference between an okay meal and a memorable one. In the kitchen, think of yourself as an artist, layering flavor, aroma, and color with every dash or sprinkle and experimenting with a multitude of options.

> **Wholesome Habits**
>
> Did you know that 75 percent of what we taste is actually a result of smell? To see, or rather smell, for yourself, slice a grapefruit and an orange in half, close your eyes, plug your nose, and take a taste of each one. You probably won't be able to distinguish between the two citrus fruits.

Herbs and spices create excitement and diversity unmatched by most other food types. Consider a simple tomato and onion mixture. Add basil and garlic to make it Italian. Toss in some cilantro and cumin for a Mexican twist. Or sprinkle it with turmeric and ginger for a taste of India. If you're unsure of what spices and herbs go together, look at the ethnic foods these seasonings are paired with. The cuisines of different countries will educate and inspire you in the art of using herbs and spices. Then let your imagination soar and tap your own creativity.

Don't Be a Salty Dog

Of all the seasonings in the world, salt is by far the most popular. Not only does it taste good on its own, it enhances the flavor of food while also preserving it. However, our dependency on salt has a price—namely, high blood pressure, heart disease, and kidney problems. Typical American intakes can reach more than 4,000 mg sodium a day—that's 75 percent higher than the 2,400 mg recommended daily intake. Clean eaters take in much less salt—probably around 1,500 mg or so daily—without even trying very hard. How can we do it?

The solution is very simple: eliminate processed food. More than three quarters of the total sodium intake in the standard American diet comes from processed foods. Most people don't even realize how much they're taking in when they eat processed food.

How often have you seen people salting their food before they even taste it? That's just wrong. Sodium is naturally found in many foods like vegetables, so it's often unnecessary to add salt. In addition, adding too much salt can mask the flavor of the food. To keep sodium in check, limit the salt you add while cooking or, better yet, don't add any at all while you're preparing the food. Then if you need to you can add salt at the end, but always taste your food first to be sure it needs it.

If you do want to sprinkle some salt on your food be sure and make it clean. Clean salt choices are natural, unrefined, and unprocessed with no added ingredients. These include kosher salt, sea salt, and specialty salts like fleur de sel, French grey sea salt, celtic sea salt, and Himalayan crystal salt.

Dirty Secrets

If you're wondering which foods provide the most sodium in the typical American diet (by how much is eaten as well as sodium content), here they are in order: meat pizza, white bread, processed cheese, hot dogs, spaghetti (refined) with sauce, ham, and store-bought ketchup. All of these foods are off-limits on the clean eating diet.

While all salt contains the same amount of sodium by weight—380 mg of sodium per gram—you may notice different sodium levels listed on the label. This is because the shape and the size of the salt crystals vary. The coarser or bigger the salt granule, the less sodium per teaspoon. For example, a ¼ teaspoon of coarse kosher salt has 480 mg of sodium, while the same amount of finely ground salt has 590 mg sodium. Shape and size also affect taste. Used as a finishing salt, big crystal salts often taste saltier because they burst on the tip of your tongue and don't easily dissolve in food.

Kick It Up a Notch

If you're looking to perk up bland tasting food, try adding some chili peppers. They're high in vitamins C and A and naturally low in calories, making them an ideal clean food. Once you get past the heat, they also boast a depth of flavor that ranges from smoky and chocolaty to sweet and fruity. Chile peppers come in all sizes, shapes, colors, and levels of heat, making them adaptable to any food or cooking style. Consider that all the major cuisines of the world include chili peppers in one form or another in their repertoire.

Be careful cutting hot peppers; capsaicin, the chemical responsible for their intense heat, can burn your hands and any other part of the body you touch, so wear plastic food handling gloves. Since most of the capsaicin is located in the ribs and seeds, removing them drastically decreases the burn.

Wholesome Habits _____

The capsaicin level, or heat index, of peppers is measured in scoville units, named after William Scoville, a pharmacist who came up with the scoring system in 1912. The units go up by factors of 10 with 0 being the mildest, sweet bell pepper and going up to hot, hot, hot. The hottest pepper in the world is the Naga Jolokia, a red pepper from India with a rating of more than 1,000,000 scoville units; next in line is the Red Savina habanero with nearly 600,000 scoville units. A jalapeño is considered a lightweight at a mere 2,500 units.

Pack It Up

In order to eat every two to three hours, it's crucial that you always keep clean food at the ready. If you're at home this shouldn't be a problem, but when you're at work or running errands all day, eating regularly and eating clean can be a challenge. Overcoming these hurdles is really just a matter of planning. Here are ways to make it work.

Breakfast Matters

You've heard it a million times before, but it's worth repeating: breakfast is the most important meal of the day! After fasting all night (while sleeping) your body needs fuel to restart its engine and get blood pumping to your heart and your brain. Aside from giving you energy, feeding your body in the A.M. clears away that morning fog, enabling you to think clearly, remember better, and concentrate so you can be at your best throughout the day. As a matter of fact, studies show that children who eat breakfast consistently perform better on cognitive tests.

Eating breakfast also does wonders for your weight. In fact, if you're trying to lose weight, eating breakfast is the way to do it. Why? It prevents you from noshing on high-calorie snacks or overeating later in the day. Not only are breakfast eaters leaner than those who opt to skip this meal, but also generally they eat fewer total calories per day. Calories eaten early in the day have another thing going for them, too: they're less likely to turn into fat than their late-night counterparts.

Dirty Secrets _____

Beware of protein bars, which are often high in fat, sugar, and calories, making them more like a glorified candy bar. In addition they're usually filled with "unclean" ingredients. Our advice, skip the bar and grab some fruit and cheese instead.

But simply grabbing a fruit snack or a piece of whole wheat toast isn't enough. You have to eat the right kind of breakfast—one that's rich in carbohydrates and protein, and low in fat. And no skimping, you should eat a big breakfast!

So what should you dine on at dawn? Anything you want, really. You can have peanut butter, an apple, milk, and a hardboiled egg; or you can have last night's dinner warmed up. You can have a bowl of oatmeal, a scrambled egg and orange juice, or a cold turkey sandwich. What's most important is that you have a good balance of nutrients and at least 300 to 400 calories. Don't worry if you're not a morning person—it doesn't take long for your stomach to adjust to the new routine. Here's how to keep breakfast on the menu everyday:

- Plan breakfast the night before.

- Freeze individual morning meals or breads, then pull them out the night before or even in the morning.

- Always keep some portable foods around, that you can take with you to the office if you're running late.

Bring a Lunch, Pack a Snack

Lunch time can also run you into trouble, especially if you go out to eat often. To help stay clean at work, start by packing a lunch most days of the week. You'll save cash as well as calories, since the cost of eating out can rack up quickly.

When preparing your lunch, be sure to include snacks as well. I've found the best way to do this is to keep snacks in separate bags, labeled A.M. and P.M. Schedule a time for snacks, too. Sometimes we get so busy that we forget to eat, which is not good for our bodies or our minds.

Keep a supply of clean snack foods at the office for emergencies. In your desk, best bets are nuts, all-natural peanut butter, dried fruit, and dry cereal. If you have access to a refrigerator, store yogurt, milk, low-fat cheese, and fruit.

If you do go out to lunch, look for self-serve salad bars and hot buffets, and be sure and tell your dining out colleagues about your clean eating lifestyle.

When Temptation Calls

Despite your best efforts, there will come a time when you're tempted to stray. Try one or more of these strategies to keep you on track:

- **Don't tempt yourself.** Stick to the mantra out-of-sight out-of mind and know the foods that you can't refuse. For example if potato chips are your downfall, don't keep any in the house. If the smell of pizza drives you crazy, change the route you take to work or school so you don't pass your favorite pizza parlor.

- **Walk away.** If you have a craving you just can't shake, take a brisk 10 minute walk outside or do a few light exercises or stretches. The activity will get your mind off the food and burn some calories as well.

- **Write it down.** Studies show people who keep a food journal lose more weight than those who don't. There's something about the act of writing down what you eat that automatically makes you become more conscientious and a better eater.

- **Turn off the TV.** When it comes to living clean, television watching is at the bottom of the list. Why? First, you are constantly bombarded with commercials for delicious-looking processed food, mainly fast food and restaurant food. Second, if you watch TV while you're eating, you're not paying attention to your food and can easily overeat. Finally, too much TV watching promotes a sedentary lifestyle, which is exactly what you are trying to avoid.

Dirty Secrets

The more television you watch (and computer games you play) the more likely you are to put on the pounds. One study found people who watched TV three hours or more a day were twice as likely to be obese than those who viewed an hour or less a day.

- **Create your own convenience foods.** I call these emergency food supplies, because when you're hungry all you have to do is pop them right in the microwave. The next time you're preparing your favorite meal, make some extra and freeze it in single serving containers. One of my specialties is vegetable lasagna, but you can also do it with chicken, beef, or pork; be sure and include sides like whole grain rice blends and vegetables. Simply put it all together as if you were going to serve yourself a complete meal. Seal, wrap, label, and freeze.

If You Get Dirty ...

Clean eating is more than a diet—it is a lifestyle—and like any lifestyle there's got to be some flexibility built in, especially for dealing with special occasions, celebrations, or even just a night out. Eating clean means eating healthy, but this doesn't mean you may never again have a Philly cheese steak or a BLT, especially if you love them. If you slip up and eat something that isn't clean, don't fret about it. Just move on and eat clean the next meal and the next.

The Cheat

The truth is, many clean eaters allow themselves one cheat meal a week where they can break the rules. Most times these meals are reserved for dining out. For people who are just starting out eating clean, this one-night-a-week cheat is a lifesaver and may even help motivate you to stay on track the other six days.

Others who are well-adjusted to the clean eating lifestyle find cravings for these highly processed foods are reduced, so many of these cheat meals may not even be real cheats at all. Rather than an indulgent meal, clean eaters may simply enjoy a piece of birthday cake or a bite or two of some special dinner. You may even find yourself skipping your cheat meal altogether. But this doesn't mean you can bank those calories and add an extra cheat meal the next week (they aren't like roll over minutes!). Unless there's a really special occasion twice in one week, try to stick with once a week.

Slow and Steady

Your goal should be to follow a healthy, processed-free diet about 80 to 90 percent of the time. If you are working out and eating clean five or six days a week, one rich meal won't make much of a difference. However, this is not a license for going completely overboard. You should watch your portion size and try to increase your intake of fruits and vegetables on your cheat day.

Eating clean means eating healthy over the long haul. So rather than focus on what you can't have, think about what you can eat. If you're having a bad day or just not really motivated, think of that old fairy tale about the turtle and the hare. Although the hare was faster, it was the slow and steady turtle who won the race.

Clean Cuts

If you want to stick to clean eating, don't eliminate the foods you love. This can set up feelings of deprivation and longing so strong they can end up sabotaging your healthy diet. Rather, incorporate favorite foods into your cheat meals. This way you can enjoy them once a week.

The Least You Need to Know

- Herbs, spices, and chile peppers offer countless ways to boost the flavor of clean eating meals without any fat, sugar, or salt.

- Salt, which is mostly found in highly refined and processed foods, is low on the clean eating regime.

- Make breakfast the most important meal of the day. It supplies you with energy and prevents you from overeating later in the day.

- Bring lunches and snacks with you when you're on the go to avoid the temptation of high-fat, high-salt fast-food meals and snacks.

- One cheat meal a week prevents you from feeling deprived and keeps you motivated for the long haul.

Chapter 5

How Clean Can You Be?

In This Chapter

- ◆ What it means to be clean and green
- ◆ The problem with plastics
- ◆ Living a wheat-free life
- ◆ Dealing with dairy

With concern over the earth's environmental resources at an all-time high, "going green" has become increasingly popular. Once considered a passing trend, the green movement has evolved into a part of mainstream culture and appears to be here to stay. "Going green" means following a healthy, environmentally sound, and sustainable lifestyle. Eating green follows many of the same principles of clean eating, only taking it one step further to include eco-friendly, organic, local foods free of pesticides and chemical fertilizers. This chapter takes a look at the issues behind eating green and what it means to be a clean green machine.

Other people take clean eating in entirely different directions. For them clean means more than just eating whole, unprocessed, unrefined foods. It also involves eliminating foods that are potentially harmful for people sensitive to food allergies or who have other health conditions.

This version of eating clean includes going wheat-free, dairy-free, or both. In this chapter we review what it takes to do both while still living the clean lifestyle.

Go Clean and Green

For some people, being clean and green is one and the same. After all, how could whole, natural foods be considered healthy if they're loaded with pesticides, chemical fertilizers, hormones, and other unnatural substances? While you don't have to eat green to eat clean, and vice versa, most clean eaters drift toward green tendencies in all aspects of their lives.

So what exactly is green cuisine? Green cuisine is food that is both healthy and environmentally friendly. It is also food that uses the least amount of energy to produce. For example, an apple takes less energy to produce than apple juice, because the juice needs to be pressed, strained, and pasteurized.

Organic foods are grown or raised without conventional pesticides, herbicides, synthetic fertilizers, growth hormones, antibiotics, or creating sewage sludge. Once produced, the food is minimally processed with no artificial ingredients or preservatives. Organic farms use *sustainable* farming practices.

> **Clean Meanings**
>
> **Sustainable** agriculture protects and replenishes the earth's natural resources. It integrates profitable farming with environmental and social consciousness by promoting continuous yet environmentally protective farming techniques.

Live like a Locavore

Locavores are people who pay attention to where their food comes from and commit to eating as many locally-grown and produced foods as possible. Buying local foods has numerous benefits. First, it supports local business and fosters closer connections to your community. Being closer to the origin of your food makes it easier to find out whether the food is clean or not. It also increases your chances that the food *will* be clean, mostly due to the fact that many small business owners are more concerned with quality than quantity and are willing to go the extra mile without adding refined or synthetic ingredients. Removing these ingredients isn't cost effective for many big businesses.

Since locally produced food doesn't have to travel far to get to your door, it burns less fossil fuel, and so contributes to the fight against global warming.

Ask any locavore why they buy their food locally, and one of their top answers will probably involve taste. Local foods simply taste better than their road-weary counterparts. Certainly, locally-grown produce is fresher than its grocery store counterpart, since it hasn't traveled thousands of miles. It also stays on the plant longer, meaning it has more time to ripen, turning starches into naturally sweet sugars. Without the pressure of producing food that has to travel long distances, farmers can experiment with a wider assortment of produce, like heirloom varieties of tomatoes, eggplants, or peppers. Fresh produce also provides a sense that the world is in a natural order. Tomatoes come out in summer, apples in fall, berries in spring. Every food has its place in the seasons.

So what does eating local have to do with health? The better the produce tastes, the more likely you are to eat it and to eat more of it, in its natural state. When it comes to fruits and vegetables—even meats, cheeses, and legumes—the fresher it is, the better it tastes. The shorter the time between when it is picked and when it is eaten the more nutritional value the produce has, adding another notch to the healthy quotient. With these points in mind, eating local can lead to a cleaner, healthier life in the long run.

> **Wholesome Habits**
>
> Before the advent of transcontinental railroads, almost everyone was a locavore. If you lived on a farm you ate the foods you grew and little else. Transcontinental railroads and the rise of big cities and sprawling suburbs after World War II transformed the way we eat, increasing the distance between the farm and the dinner table. Today that tide is changing once again, and you can be a part of it.

Organic for All

One of the best things you can do for yourself, your family, and your community is to eat local and organic whenever possible. Organic farmers must adhere to strict rules regarding pesticide and fertilizer use (only organic, natural ones are allowed). This ensures you and your family are not exposed to harmful chemicals or food contaminated with pesticide residue. Gentle farming practices significantly reduce and may even eliminate pollution altogether, keeping our waterways safe and our Earth a cleaner place. More sustainable crop management builds healthy soil, which turns out stronger, sturdier plants (with more phytochemicals) and a farm that will continue to abundantly produce for many years to come. Farming this way protects our farmland as well as the farmers who work the land.

To get the USDA organic seal, farms have to be certified and regularly inspected by the USDA. They also have to follow strict plans and procedures. On packaged foods you'll see organic listed one of three ways:

- ♦ **100 percent organic:** contains 100 percent organic ingredients

- ♦ **Organic:** contains at least 95 percent organic ingredients

- ♦ **Made with organic ingredients:** contains at least 70 percent organic ingredients

Clean Cuts

To determine whether something is organic look for the USDA organic seal. If you can't find it on your fruits and veggies check the sticker. If the PLU code begins with 9 it's organic; if it begins with 4 it's conventional.

A common complaint about organic food is that it tends to cost more than conventional food. Although this is usually true, organic is worth the splurge. What better way to get fresh, pesticide free produce that tastes great? Plus, by supporting organic agriculture you can also help reduce tax dollars spent on cleaning up the problems conventional agriculture leaves behind. Think of it as an investment in your and your children's future.

Growing organic produce is more expensive because organic growers are usually smaller, and so they can't spread costs as readily as mega-factory farms. In addition, organic farming is usually more time- and labor-intensive. Finally, organic farming isn't government subsidized the way conventional farming is.

Fortunately, it's possible to be on a budget and still buy organic. All you have to do is remember these cost-saving tips:

- ♦ **Shop around.** Sometimes natural food chain stores have better prices than conventional ones.

- ♦ **Buy in season.** This could actually save you money, particularly if you are dealing with a farmer that has had a bumper crop.

- ♦ **Buy in bulk whenever possible.** Look for items sold in bulk bins at the natural foods store or stock up on sales.

- ♦ **Join a CSA (Community Supported Agriculture).** This allows you to invest in local farmers and, in return, you get a box of weekly produce from their harvest.

- ♦ **Consider buying from local farmers or ranchers even if they aren't certified organic.** Many small operations practice organic methods, but can't afford to become certified. They often advertise their produce as being pesticide free.

The Dirty Dozen

Few people can afford to go 100 percent organic. That's okay, because you really don't have to. Foods like bananas, avocadoes, mangoes, pineapple, onions, kiwi, and papaya are protected from pests and pesticides by their tough, inedible skin. This outer layer prevents pesticides from penetrating the edible interior. Other foods that face fewer threats from insects and disease (and so are sprayed less) and rank low on the amount of pesticide residues they typically contain include broccoli, cabbage, and asparagus. Buying conventionally grown versions of these foods poses little problem. Since bacteria and toxins on the outside can only get inside when you cut the produce. This is why you should always wash your produce first—yes, even those with skin—before handling.

Dirty Secrets

Just because a food says it's organic doesn't necessarily mean the food keeps you safer from food borne illness than conventional produce. The 2008 salmonella outbreak in peanuts took place in a certified organic plant.

So when does it pay to purchase organic? When growers typically apply large amounts of pesticides, inject the livestock with hormones, use a lot of additives, or when the food or fruit readily traps these chemicals, such as in the crevices of raspberries or blackberries. The Environmental Working Group (EWG), a nonprofit consumer activist group based in Washington, D.C., regularly puts together a list of the top "dirty dozen" fruits and vegetables, ranking foods based on the amount of pesticide residues they contain. According to EWG, you can cut your total exposure as much as 90 percent by spending your organic dollars on the most contaminated produce. Here is EWG's list of dirtiest produce, starting with the dirtiest:

1. Peaches
2. Apples
3. Sweet bell peppers
4. Celery
5. Nectarines
6. Strawberries
7. Cherries
8. Pears
9. Grapes (imported)
10. Spinach
11. Lettuce
12. Potatoes

What about Meat, Poultry, and Dairy?

Always try to purchase organic meat, poultry, and dairy. In addition to being healthier for your own body, organic meat is healthier for the environment.

Organic ranchers practice earth-friendly sustainable practices that have less impact on the environment and use less energy. To be in compliance, animals are treated humanely and are given no growth hormones or antibiotics (except to treat a sick animal). Livestock must be fed 100 percent organic feed with no animal by-products, and the animals must spend time outdoors in the fresh air.

On labels or menus you'll often see organic meats labeled as "free-range" or "ranch-raised." This is a tip off that the animals were raised more humanely.

"Grass-fed" is another green light word worth looking for. Ranchers can call their meat grass-fed only if the animal was raised on a diet of 100 percent grass and forage (no grain) with continuous access to pasture most of the season. Compared to grain-fed beef, grass-fed beef is healthier and better for you. It contains higher levels of omega-3 fats, good fats known to reduce heart disease risk, and lower levels of total fat.

Although pricey, organic milk is another option worth considering, especially if you drink a lot of milk or have small children. By law, organic milk comes from cows not treated with artificial growth hormones such as *recombinant bovine somatotropin (rBST)* and antibiotics. Cows also must eat feed grown without pesticides and have access to pasture.

Dirty Secrets _____

Some meat is labeled as "grass-fed, grain finished," meaning the cows were given grain the last few months before processing, basically to fatten them up. However, grain-finished beef changes the composition of the meat and makes it more like conventional meat. Given the choice, always choose 100 percent grass-fed.

Clean Meanings _____

Recombinant bovine somatotropin (rBST) is a man-made growth hormone used to increase milk production in cows. Animal welfare experts say cows treated with rBST have weaker bones (resulting in lameness) and are more susceptible to infections. More infections, means the cow must be treated with more antibiotics fostering concern about new strains of antibiotic resistant bacteria. In humans, some studies show rBST may increase cancer risk. And, although the FDA says there's no difference between rBST-treated and non-rBST-treated cows, many conventional dairies no longer use it. Unfortunately not all conventional artificial hormone-free milk is labeled. So, for now your best bet for insuring you don't get milk from rBST treated cows is to buy certified organic.

Bye Bye Biotechnology

Biotechnology is the science of altering an animal or plant's makeup through genetic modification. Typically this involves introducing a gene from one species or organism into another. Many people are concerned that biotechnology will have long-term negative effects on our environment, our health, and our food supply. These genetic traits are handed down from generation to generation. Fortunately, the USDA's organic label guarantees you won't be eating any of the following types of genetically altered foods:

◆ **Genetically modified organisms (GMO).** GMOs are found primarily in plants. GMO plants have had their genes altered to improve production, resist disease, and otherwise "improve" a crop. Some people estimate as much as 70 percent of our grocery food contains GMO, thanks mostly to the prevalence of genetically modified soy and corn in processed foods. Produce with stickers that begin with the PLU number 8 are GMO.

◆ **Genetically engineered animals.** These animals have snippets of DNA from other animals, plants, or organisms inserted into their genes, such as a pig with a fish gene to increase omega-3 content in the meat.

◆ **Cloned meat and milk.** This comes from cloned cattle, pig, and goats and their offspring.

Beware of BPA

Part of the clean green lifestyle is cooking more and eating out less. This often means bringing food stored in plastic containers with you to work, sporting events, even to the gym. Although authorities tell us that most plastics are safe, one chemical, called bisphenol-A (BPA), has caused a great deal of concern among health authorities. This chemical is found in hard, clear plastic; plastic bottles with the number 7 on the bottom are likely to contain BPA.

BPA can leach into food and beverages, and continuous low-level exposure is thought to increase your risk of heart disease, cancer, and obesity. The Centers for Disease Control first brought attention to this issue in 2005, and many manufacturers now make BPA-free plastic containers, cups, and bottles. Even so, it's a good idea to avoid putting plastics in the dishwasher or microwave, as high temperatures can cause deterioration and more BPA to leach out. Other tips—toss out old, worn, or stained plastics as this indicates the plastic is breaking down and more BPA will be released. Other plastics to avoid include those with the recycling numbers 3 and 6.

Be Free

Sometimes people choose to eat clean for medical reasons such as health or gastrointestinal problems. Most often this involves an allergy, intolerance, or health condition. These individuals often modify their clean diet to exclude such items as wheat or dairy in addition to the other principles we've discussed. Since people who are sensitive to wheat are more likely to have trouble with dairy as well, there's also a clean wheat-free and dairy-free diet.

Why Go Wheat-Free

With the exception of those with a wheat allergy, which is generally detected in children under three and affects only a small percentage of the population, most people who decide to eat a clean wheat-free diet have probably been experiencing problems with wheat for a while. These people generally fall into two camps—those who have specific gluten sensitivity known as celiac disease, and those who just can't tolerate wheat.

Celiac disease is a genetic autoimmune disorder in which gluten, a protein found in wheat, causes your body to attack the small intestine, blocking absorption and causing a host of problems. Although most symptoms center around the digestive system—like bloating, gas, cramps, and diarrhea—people with celiac disease may also suffer skin rashes, headaches, sinus infections, fatigue, infertility, and more. The severity of the symptoms varies widely from very mild to debilitating sickness. Recent strides in recognizing the illness has caused a surge of cases, making us think it's much more common than previously thought. Experts say celiac affects as many as 3 million Americans.

Wholesome Habits

Surprisingly in Italy, a nation known for its great pasta dishes, celiac disease occurs in about 1 in every 250 people. It's so common that all Italian children are routinely screened for the condition by age 6.

People with wheat intolerances experience some of the same symptoms as celiacs, except the gluten does not trigger an immune response. Like people with celiac disease, the only way to get rid of offending symptoms is to remove the culprit—wheat and/or gluten—and the only way most people know if they really are sensitive to wheat is to go on a wheat-free diet and see how they feel. Other people who might do well avoiding gluten and wheat include those with multiple sclerosis, rheumatoid arthritis, lupus, autism, and asthma. As much as 15 percent of the American population could suffer from some type of wheat intolerance or gluten sensitivity (celiac disease).

Taking the Plunge

If you already eat clean, making the wheat-free plunge isn't as hard as you may think. The bulk of your diet—fresh whole fruits, vegetables, meats, and legumes—is naturally wheat-free. You've also cut out fatty breads and fried foods, another place where gluten sneaks in. For some people the most troublesome part of going gluten-free is watching out for hidden gluten found in processed, packaged, and frozen foods. But you're already ahead of the game here, too.

You need to pay attention to breads, cereals, and grain-based dishes. Going wheat-free means eliminating all wheat, barley, rye, and oats. (Technically, oats do not contain gluten, but because the machines used to process oats typically do, people with gluten intolerances often avoid them. Gluten-free oats are now available.) Other kinds of wheat to watch out for are wheat berries, spelt, triticale, faro, malt kamut, and bulgur.

Don't be put off by this list. Increased consumer demand has generated dozens of gluten-free products. Look around and you'll find a wealth of food choices.

Aside from corn and rice, other gluten-free grains include amaranth, buckwheat, millet, sorghum, quinoa, teff, and specialty flours (check out some of the nut and legume flours now available). Some mainstream stores have dedicated whole sections to gluten-free living, so you might not even have to go to a specialty store to find what you are looking for.

The Dairy Dilemma

Wheat and dairy intolerances often go hand in hand. No one really knows why this is the case, except that perhaps people with these intolerances are just more sensitive to all kinds of foods.

Lactose is a natural sugar found in cow's milk. People who have trouble digesting milk and milk products are called lactose intolerant. They lack an enzyme called lactase, which breaks down lactose in the body. As newborns we produce loads of lactase so we can easily drink mother's milk, but as we age and milk becomes less important to our diet, our lactase levels change. By age 5, lactase levels drop off sharply. People who drink milk and eat dairy regularly rarely suffer any consequences, mostly because their bodies adapt. Bacteria, which naturally live in your gut, take up where lactase leaves off and neutralize milk sugar. Making sure you always eat dairy along with other foods also lessens the likelihood you will experience any symptoms.

Since dairy foods can be high in fat, giving them up will help you slim down and become leaner. Weight loss is one of the main reasons why people cut dairy out of their diet. Dairy products can also rack up sodium levels quickly, which is another reason why clean eaters limit their intake.

Unless you have a milk allergy (which means all milk products are always off-limits), going dairy-free doesn't have to be an all-or-nothing proposition. Even people with dairy intolerances can usually tolerate small amounts of yogurt or aged cheese. The point is to give yourself and your body a break from eating dairy foods every day. The change will do you good.

> ### Clean Cuts
>
> If you are considering cutting down or eliminating dairy from your diet, here's another thing to think about: dairy foods are rich sources of bone-building nutrients, such as calcium, phosphorus, and vitamins A and D. If you're concerned about getting enough of those nutrients, choose fortified soymilk, orange juice, or rice milk and up your intake of green vegetables, sardines, and salmon.

Rising to the Challenge

Deciding to eat clean and dairy-free is more than just taking the cheese out of your diet. It also means getting rid of butter, cream, sour cream, milk, and yogurt, as well as those foods containing hidden milk products such as lactose, casein, whey, and milk solids that can be found in foods like canned tuna, chicken broth, and bread. Here are a few tips to keep you on track.

Turn to soy. Soy products can often replace the creamy texture and consistency of dairy foods. Best bets to try are unsweetened or vanilla flavored soymilk, soy ice cream (coconut ice cream is another nondairy ice cream worth trying), soy yogurt, and soy cheese. Tofu is another option. I call it the great pretender because it takes on whatever flavor it's paired with, adding body and substance.

Pump up flavor with herbs and spices. On the clean eating regime, cheese is often sprinkled on as a finishing touch to boost flavor. In restaurants, chefs have a reputation for being heavy handed with butter and cream for the same reason. Instead of dairy, add a dash of flavor with a sprinkle of fresh herbs or a drizzle of flavored olive oil. Just keep in mind that a little goes a long way.

The Least You Need to Know

◆ The best way to eat clean and green is to buy organic, locally grown produce, meat, and dairy as much as possible.

◆ Use only BPA-free plastic.

◆ People with gluten intolerance should exclude all wheat, barley, oats, rye, spelt, and bulgur from their diet.

◆ If you're already eating a clean diet, eliminating dairy is easy.

Part 2

Jump-Start Your Morning

The world can generally be divided into two camps: breakfast eaters and breakfast skippers. My husband is a breakfast eater and, before I started eating clean, I was a breakfast skipper. Now that I've opened my eyes to the morning meal, I have a lot more energy during the day and even find myself eating less overall throughout the day.

You cannot overestimate the power of a good breakfast. In Part 2, you'll learn how to prepare an assortment of nutritious morning meals, including hot and cold cereals; smoothies; egg dishes; and breads, muffins, and pancakes. All clean, all healthful, all natural, and all delicious.

Some of these recipes, like the Fabulous Fruit Smoothie, can be whipped up in a flash for a quick weekday breakfast. Others, such as Zucchini-Carrot Bread, are best prepared the night before. Still others—Orange Buckwheat Pancakes come to mind—make wonderful leisurely Sunday morning meals.

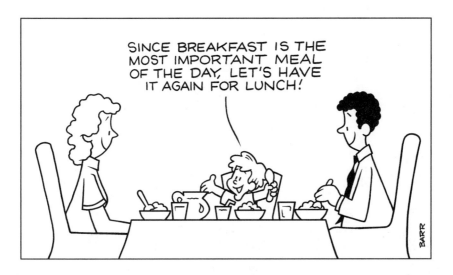

Chapter 6

Quick Starts

In This Chapter

- ◆ Oatmeal like you've never eaten it before
- ◆ Eye-opening breakfast cereal blends
- ◆ Satisfying smoothies

Breakfast cereals have a lot of things going for them. They're fast, easy to eat, typically high in fiber, and well-endowed with plenty of vitamins and minerals. Unfortunately, most store-bought brands are highly processed and loaded with sugar (especially high-fructose corn syrup). And with a list of ingredients an arm's length long, it just might take you longer to read the side of the box than it does to eat a bowl of what's inside.

That's why homemade cereals are the way to go for clean eaters. This chapter offers up several hot and cold recipes we think you'll like so much you'll prepare them again and again. They're chock full of nuts, seeds, whole grains, and fresh or dried fruit.

Each one of these morning meals is filling and satisfying, but they're also wholesome, nourishing, and packed with good-for-you-nutrients like B vitamins, iron, magnesium, and selenium.

Since we know time is the biggest barrier for eating breakfast, we made sure that most of these hot cereals come together in minutes. The two cold cereals—our Multigrain Cold Cereal Blend and Tropical Kasha Cereal Blend—are best prepared ahead of time, but once made they make a great grab-and-go breakfast during the week.

If you're one of those people who are always running late or if you're just not a "cereal-kind-of-person," we've got you covered with a bevy of great breakfast smoothies. Prepared the night before or whipped up in a blender that morning, who can resist meals in a glass like Peaches and Cream Smoothie or Fabulous Fruit Smoothie. You'll be surprised at just how fast and delicious a healthy breakfast can be.

Honey Date Porridge

Inspired by the wonderful cornmeal polentas of northern Italy, this sweet hot cereal is flecked with chopped dates and drizzled with honey and toasted walnuts. It's sweet enough to be a dessert but filling enough to be a meal.

1 cup unsweetened soymilk	**1 tsp. honey**
⅓ to ½ cup water	**3 tsp. chopped walnuts, toasted**
½ cup whole stone-ground cornmeal	**Dash allspice**
3 small dates, chopped	

Yield: 4 servings
Prep time: 5 minutes
Cook time: 10 minutes
Serving size: ¾ cup
Each serving has:
209 calories
5 g total fat
1 g saturated fat
7 g protein
36 g carbohydrate
11 g sugars
0 mg cholesterol
4 g fiber
46 mg sodium

1. Bring soymilk and water to a boil in a medium saucepot over medium-high heat. Slowly pour cornmeal in a continuous stream into boiling water, while beating vigorously with a wooden spoon to prevent any lumps from forming.

2. Lower the heat and keep beating cornmeal until smooth, about 1 or 2 minutes, until it begins to boil. Mix in chopped dates, cook for another minute. Remove from heat.

3. To serve, place ¾ cup porridge in each bowl, drizzle with ¼ teaspoon honey, ¾ teaspoon chopped nuts, and a dash of allspice. Serve warm.

Clean Cuts

Stone-ground cornmeal is your best bet because it contains the whole grain, including the germ. Other kinds of processing remove the germ. Stone-ground cornmeal is available in yellow, white, or blue varieties, depending on the type of corn.

Sweet Potato Flaxseed Oatmeal

Sweet potato, oatmeal, and flaxseed might sound like an unusual combination, particularly for breakfast, but once you've tasted it you'll be sold. Sweet potato pairs beautifully with maple syrup and cinnamon and, when blended with oatmeal, creates a sweet, memorable, morning meal.

To save time, bake your sweet potato ahead of time. When cool, wrap it tightly and freeze it. Then all you need to do is thaw the potato, mash it, and mix it in. Leftover mashed sweet potatoes will also work well in this recipe.

Yield: 4 servings
Prep time: 5 minutes
Cook time: 5 minutes
Serving size: ¾ cup
Each serving has:
183 calories
4 g total fat
0 g saturated fat
5 g protein
33 g carbohydrate
6 g sugars
0 mg cholesterol
5 g fiber
17 mg sodium

3 cups water

1½ cups old-fashioned rolled oats

1 small sweet potato, cooked and mashed

4 tsp. ground flaxseed

3 tsp. maple syrup

½ tsp. ground cinnamon

2 tsp. chopped pecans

1. Bring water to a boil in a small saucepot over medium-high heat. Mix in oatmeal and cook for 3 minutes. Add mashed sweet potato, flaxseed, 1 teaspoon maple syrup, and cinnamon. Blend and simmer 2 or 3 more minutes.

2. To serve, top each ¾ cup portion with ½ teaspoon of remaining maple syrup and ½ teaspoon chopped pecans. Serve immediately.

Wholesome Habits

Although the terms *sweet potato* and *yam* are used interchangeably in U.S. markets, they are very distinct vegetables. Sweet potatoes are moist and sweet with an orange flesh and thin skin. Yams are starchier, like potatoes, and have a creamy or white flesh with a rough, scaly dark brown skin. Most produce labeled yams in the United States are actually a variety of sweet potato.

Orange Oatmeal Crème Brulee

In this special-occasion breakfast treat, wholesome oatmeal is topped with orange sections then layered with creamy custard. The result is a rich and filling breakfast you won't believe is clean and nutritious, much less only 137 calories per serving.

4 cups water

2½ cups old-fashioned rolled oats

Pinch salt

1 cup low-fat (1 percent) milk

2 cups evaporated whole milk

2 whole large eggs

1 large egg white

½ cup Sucanat

1 tsp. vanilla extract

Juice of 1 orange (about ¼ cup)

Zest of 1 orange (about 2 tsp.)

Sections of 2 oranges, cut into ½-inch pieces

¼ tsp. ground cinnamon

Yield: 16 servings
Prep time: 25 minutes
Cook time: 25 minutes
Serving size: ½ cup
Each serving has:
137 calories
4 g total fat
2 g saturated fat
6 g protein
20 g carbohydrate
6 g sugars
36 mg cholesterol
2 g fiber
70 mg sodium

1. Heat the oven to 425°F. Heat water to boiling in a medium-size saucepot. Mix in oats and salt and simmer for 5 minutes. Set aside.

2. In another saucepot heat low-fat milk and evaporated milk until bubbles form around the edges. Milk should be scalding hot but not boiling.

3. Beat whole eggs, egg white, Sucanat, and vanilla in a small bowl. Slowly mix in hot milk, whisking mixture while pouring. Add orange juice, orange zest, and cinnamon.

4. Spray a 9×13-inch pan with cooking spray. Spread oatmeal in an even layer on the bottom of the pan. Sprinkle orange wedges evenly over top. Pour milk mixture over oatmeal and oranges. Place pan in oven and bake for 25 minutes. Custard will be firm but still jiggles slightly. Let sit for 10 to 15 minutes. Cut and serve warm or hot.

Variation: You can replace the bottom layer with any other thick hot cereal or cooked grain, such as grits or cream of wheat. Or you can create your own oatmeal blend. Consider this option: Boil 2¾ cups water, then add 1¾ cups oatmeal and 2 tablespoons ground flaxseed. Cook for about 3 to 4 minutes. Mix in ½ cup cooked amaranth. Cook another 1 or 2 minutes.

Wholesome Habits

Amaranth is a nutritional powerhouse grain native to the Andes mountains. Its tiny beige or black grains stay on the crunchy side even after cooking. It has a grassy, earthy flavor that works well in porridges. To cook, bring 3¼ cups water to boil and whisk in 1 cup amaranth. Return to a boil, cover, reduce heat to simmer, and cook for 20 to 25 minutes. Add water if grain begins to stick to bottom of pot. Amaranth will be soft but still crunchy. It's great when reheated.

Multigrain Cold Cereal Blend

This cold cereal blend featuring cooked brown rice, millet, wheat berries, and barley tastes even better the next day, when the grains have softened and had a chance to absorb the honey. Although I included it in the breakfast chapter, it's excellent any time of day.

6 cups water

½ cup short grain brown rice

½ cup wheat berries

½ cup pearled barley

¼ cup millet

1 tsp. ground cinnamon

2 TB. maple syrup

½ cup chopped walnuts, toasted

Yield: 8 servings
Prep time: 20 minutes
Cook time: 50 minutes, plus draining and drying time (2¼ hours)
Serving size: ¾ cup
Each serving has:
210 calories
6 g total fat
1 g saturated fat
5 g protein
37 g carbohydrate
4 g sugars
0 mg cholesterol
5 g fiber
2 mg sodium

1. In a 4-quart pot heat 5¼ cups water over medium-high heat. When water boils add brown rice, wheat berries, and barley. Return to a boil, reduce heat to simmer, and cover. Simmer for 45 to 50 minutes, until grains are tender. Add water as necessary.

2. While grains are cooking, bring ¾ cup water to boil. In separate small saucepot pour in dry millet and heat over medium-high heat for 4 to 6 minutes or until it becomes toasty brown and smells like popcorn (watch out—it may begin to pop), stirring constantly. When millet has browned pour in boiling water, being careful to avoid splattering. Reduce heat to simmer, cover, and cook for 15 to 18 minutes. If the millet begins to stick, add more water. It should be light and fluffy looking. Spoon cooked millet into a bowl and set aside.

3. When rice mixture is done, remove from heat and put in strainer to drain. Drain for 15 minutes.

4. In large bowl gently mix drained grains and millet with a wooden spoon. Add cinnamon, maple syrup, and walnuts and mix. Evenly spread grains on 2 baking sheets and let air dry for 2 hours.

5. Serve with milk or yogurt or store in an airtight container in the refrigerator. Grain mixture will keep in the refrigerator for a week or you can freeze it for up to 3 months.

Clean Cuts

To toast nuts, place them in a small dry skillet and heat over medium heat, tossing constantly, until they are slightly brown and smell nutty, about 5 to 7 minutes. Another option is to place nuts in an even layer in a small shallow pan and toast in a preheated 350°F oven for 10 to 15 minutes, stirring frequently. Toasting intensifies "nutty" flavor and crunchiness.

Tropical Kasha Cereal Blend

Cooked *kasha* adds another flavor dimension to the Multigrain Cold Cereal Blend in this sweet version, flavored with mango, coconut, and banana. Make a double batch as it's sure to go fast.

½ cup water

¼ cup whole grain kasha

3 cups Multigrain Cold Cereal Blend (see recipe earlier in this chapter)

½ cup mango, small diced

2 TB. shredded coconut, unsweetened

1 small banana, chopped

Yield: 5 servings	
Prep time: 5 minutes	
Cook time: 10 minutes plus ½ hour drying time	
Serving size: ¾ cup	
Each serving has:	
242 calories	
6 g total fat	
1 g saturated fat	
5 g protein	
44 g carbohydrate	
9 g sugars	
0 mg cholesterol	
6 g fiber	
4 mg sodium	

1. Heat water over medium-high heat until boiling. Add kasha, lower the heat to a simmer, and cook, covered, for 10 minutes. Stir occasionally.

2. When kasha is cooked, spread onto a baking sheet in an even layer to dry for ½ hour. When cool, mix kasha, cereal blend, mango, coconut, and banana together.

3. Serve immediately. If not serving immediately omit the banana and store in airtight container in the refrigerator. Mixture will keep in refrigerator for up to a week.

Variation: You can use almost any type of fruit mixture in this cereal blend.

Clean Meanings

Kasha is the Eastern European name for toasted buckwheat groats (groats are simply any hulled grain). You can usually find it in supermarkets where kosher products are sold. It is available fine, medium, coarsely ground, or whole.

Peaches and Cream Smoothie

Light, fruity peaches are a natural with creamy soymilk in this refreshing summer drink. Adding a touch of vanilla makes the peach flavor pop even more.

Yield: 3 servings
Prep time: 5 minutes
Serving size: 1 8-ounce cup
Each serving has:
101 calories
3 g total fat
0 g saturated fat
6 g protein
16 g carbohydrate
14 g sugars
0 mg cholesterol
2 g fiber
47 mg sodium

2 cups frozen peach slices

2 cups unsweetened soymilk

2 tsp. honey

½ tsp. vanilla or ¼ tsp. cinnamon

1. Place peaches, soymilk, honey, and vanilla in a food processor. Process on high for about 1 minute. Pour into tall glasses and serve.

Variation: You can use almost any frozen fruit for this drink. Some that work best are bananas, strawberries, mangos, and blueberries.

Clean Cuts

Frozen peaches are readily available at grocery stores, but if you want to freeze your own, just peel, pit, and slice peaches, and place them in a single layer on a cookie sheet (make sure pieces are not touching). Sprinkle peaches with lemon juice and put cookie sheet in the freezer. Once frozen, remove peaches from sheet and store in a plastic freezer bag.

Blueberry Antioxidant Smoothie

Cold, refreshing, and incredibly delicious, this creamy blueberry smoothie also has a good dose of fiber.

1 cup frozen blueberries

½ cup nonfat, plain Greek yogurt

2 TB. toasted wheat germ

1 cup unsweetened soymilk

½ TB. honey

¼ tsp. vanilla extract

Pinch cinnamon

Yield: *2 servings*
Prep time: 5 minutes
Serving size: 1 cup
Each serving has:
153 calories
3 g total fat
0 g saturated fat
12 g protein
22 g carbohydrate
16 g sugars
0 mg cholesterol
3 g fiber
60 mg sodium

1. Place all ingredients in a blender. Blend on high (purée) for about 2 minutes until smooth and creamy. Serve immediately.

Variation: You can blend almost any berry or combination of berries for this smoothie. Try strawberries, raspberries, black berries, or any combination of the three.

Clean Cuts

Frozen blueberries make this smoothie icy cold and refreshing. Don't bother buying store-bought berries; instead, simply freeze fresh ones for about ½ hour before using. Better yet, when blueberries are in season, freeze them right in their containers, wrapped tightly with plastic wrap. This way you can have fresh blueberries all year long.

Pineapple Mango Smoothie

If you don't have time for breakfast grab a glass of this pineapple mango smoothie—it's filling, sweet, and delicious.

Yield: 4 servings
Prep time: 10 minutes
Serving size: 1 cup
Each serving has:
88 calories
1 g total fat
0 g saturated fat
5 g protein
16 g carbohydrate
13 g sugars
0 mg cholesterol
1 g fiber
31 mg sodium

1 cup fresh pineapple, cut in chunks

½ mango, peeled, pitted, and coarsely chopped

½ cup nonfat, plain Greek yogurt

2 cups ice

½ cup pineapple juice

1 cup unsweetened soymilk

1. Place all ingredients in a blender, purée for about 1 minute, pulsing every 15 seconds, until smooth and frothy.

2. Serve immediately or store in an airtight container in the refrigerator for later.

Clean Cuts

Unsweetened soymilk lacks lactose, a natural sugar found in milk, so it's good for people with lactose intolerance. It also is low in sugar, containing only 2 grams per serving compared to 12 to 13 grams found in milk.

Fabulous Fruit Smoothie

Frozen fruit and soymilk make this smoothie exceptionally light, as well as quick and easy—a perfect summertime treat.

2 cups frozen mixed fruit (strawberries, peaches, pineapple, honeydew melon, and grapes)

1 cup water

1 cup pineapple juice

1 cup unsweetened soymilk

2 tsp. vanilla extract

Yield: 4 servings
Prep time: 5 minutes
Serving size: 1 cup
Each serving has:
78 calories
1 g total fat
0 g saturated fat
2 g protein
15 g carbohydrate
12 g sugars
0 mg cholesterol
1 g fiber
15 mg sodium

1. Place all ingredients in a blender. Blend on high (purée) for about 2 minutes, until smooth and creamy. Serve immediately.

 Clean Cuts

If you want to use fresh instead of frozen fruit, replace half the water with ice cubes and process the same way.

Chapter 7

Excellent Egg Dishes: Omelettes, Quiches, and More

In This Chapter

♦ Easy ways to clean up your eggs

♦ Eggs with main dish appeal—morning, noon, and night

♦ Favorite veggie combinations

The incredible, edible egg plays a major role in the clean eating diet, mostly because it's an excellent source of protein. It's the best source of protein there is, in fact. While most of this protein is found in the white, there's still a lot to be said for the yolk. Egg yolks are chock-full of vitamins and minerals like vitamins A, D, E, and K plus zinc, copper, calcium, and B vitamins. You might have heard egg yolks are high in fat, and that's true. But two thirds of that fat is the good kind. To keep your fat and calories under control, the recipes in this chapter use two or three egg whites for every yolk. This way you still get the good-for-you-nutrients, but without as much fat.

Eggs are also incredibly versatile. In this chapter we've taken the savory route and paired eggs with vegetables, bread, potatoes, and a little bit of cheese for meals that can be eaten any time of day. Any of the following recipes can be mixed and matched with your favorite vegetables, herbs, or spices. In fact, there really isn't a food eggs don't go with.

The best part is, it doesn't take much to become an egg extraordinaire in the kitchen. All you need is some creativity and imagination. So whether you want to make a simple scrambled egg or tackle a more complicated dish, we've given you some great recipes to give it a try.

Clean Broccoli Quiche

This quiche is chock full of healthful broccoli. To give it some kick we've added onions and garlic. The whole wheat bread crust not only gives it substance but rounds out the flavor, making this dish a hearty meal.

1½ cups whole wheat or multigrain bread, cut into 1-inch cubes

1 tsp. olive oil

2 TB. water

2 large eggs

4 large egg whites

1 garlic clove, peeled and minced

¼ cup onion, diced

¾ cup evaporated skim milk

¼ cup nonfat plain yogurt

¼ tsp. kosher salt

⅛ tsp. ground nutmeg

¼ tsp. black pepper

1½ cups cooked broccoli, chopped into 1-inch pieces

½ cup sharp cheddar cheese, shredded

Yield: 6 servings
Prep time: 20 minutes
Cook time: 40 minutes
Serving size: ⅙ piece
Each serving has:
202 calories
6 g total fat
3 g saturated fat
14 g protein
25 g carbohydrate
6 g sugars
82 mg cholesterol
2 g fiber
429 mg sodium

1. Preheat the oven to 425°F. Lightly spray an 8½-inch round glass pie dish with cooking spray.

2. Place bread, olive oil, and water in the food processor. Pulse until well blended and chopped into uniform pea-size pieces.

3. Press bread mixture into the bottom and sides of the pie plate to form a crust. Bake for 10 minutes or until lightly browned. Remove from oven and set aside. Lower oven temperature to 350°F.

4. In a medium bowl, whisk together eggs, egg whites, garlic, onion, evaporated milk, yogurt, salt, nutmeg, and pepper. Mix in chopped broccoli.

5. Pour broccoli-egg mixture over crust and sprinkle with shredded cheese. Bake for 35 to 40 minutes or until quiche is set. Let rest for 5 minutes. Cut into 6 pieces. Serve immediately.

Wholesome Habits

Among vegetables, broccoli tops the list for its disease-fighting powers. In various studies, broccoli has been shown to protect against stomach ulcers, heart disease, stroke, and colon and prostate cancer. Its disease-fighting power is mostly thanks to its high levels of a phytochemical called sulforaphane. Ounce for ounce, broccoli has more vitamin C than an orange and as much calcium as a glass of milk.

Potato Herb Omelet

The fresh herbs in this omelet make this dish a winner, adding color as well as taste and giving potatoes and egg a new twist. Try to use fresh herbs for this dish if you can.

1 tsp. olive oil

1 cup potato, peeled and diced into ⅜-inch pieces

1 tsp. garlic, chopped (1 small clove)

1 TB. onion, diced

1 large egg

3 large egg whites

2 TB. cold water

1 tsp. fresh marjoram leaves, finely chopped or ⅓ tsp. dried

1 tsp. fresh thyme leaves, finely chopped or ⅓ tsp. dried

1 TB. fresh parsley, finely chopped or 1 tsp. dried

¼ tsp. ground black pepper

¼ tsp. kosher salt (optional)

Yield: 1 omelet
Prep time: 15 minutes
Cook time: 10 minutes
Serving size: 1 omelet
Each serving has:
274 calories
10 g total fat
2 g saturated fat
20 g protein
29 g carbohydrate
3 g sugars
211 mg cholesterol
4 g fiber
247 mg sodium

1. Heat oil in a 10-inch skillet over medium heat. Add potato and cover, stirring frequently for about 4 minutes. Add garlic and onion, cover and cook for 2 or 3 minutes until all vegetables are soft and brown.

2. In a small bowl beat eggs, water, marjoram, thyme, parsley, pepper, and salt (if using). Pour over vegetables in skillet, cover and cook for about 3 minutes until egg puffs up. Flip omelete over and cook another minute or two. Serve immediately.

Variation: Use any combination of fresh herbs for this dish. Pick what's in season and fresh.

Clean Cuts

Using fresh herbs makes a world of difference in your cooking. To keep them fresh for as long as possible, treat them as you would fresh flowers. Snip off the ends, put them in a glass of water, cover the top with a plastic bag, and place the herbs in the refrigerator. Change the water every few days. Your herbs should last two weeks or longer.

Fajita Breakfast Wrap

Spice up your breakfast with these delicious hand-held breakfast wraps loaded with chili, eggs, peppers, onions, and a cilantro-yogurt dressing. Once you taste them we're sure you'll add them to your regular menu for breakfast, lunch, or dinner.

Yield: 2 servings
Prep time: 15 minutes
Cook time: 10 minutes
Serving size: 1 wrap
Each serving has:
247 calories
7 g total fat
1 g saturated fat
13 g protein
35 g carbohydrate
7 g sugars
106 mg cholesterol
5 g fiber
455 mg sodium

1 tsp. olive oil

½ cup onion, sliced

1 garlic clove, peeled and minced

½ cup yellow pepper, sliced

½ cup red pepper, sliced

½ cup green pepper, sliced

1 tsp. fresh cilantro, finely chopped

2 TB. nonfat plain yogurt

1 large egg

2 large egg whites

½ tsp. chili powder

1 TB. cold water

¼ tsp. kosher salt (optional)

⅛ tsp. ground black pepper

2 (8-inch) whole wheat tortillas

1. Heat oil in a 10-inch skillet over medium heat. Add onion, garlic, and peppers. Cover and let cook, stirring frequently, for about 5 minutes. Remove vegetables from skillet and put in bowl to keep warm.

2. In a small bowl whisk together cilantro and yogurt. Set aside.

3. In another small bowl whisk together eggs, chili powder, water, salt (if using), and black pepper. Lightly spray with oil the same skillet you cooked peppers in. Heat over medium heat until hot. Add egg mixture and scramble until cooked, about 2 minutes.

4. To serve, spread 1 tablespoon of cilantro sauce down the center of each tortilla. Place half of egg mixture on top, followed by half of pepper mixture. Fold the sides in about 2 inches and roll up tortilla. Serve immediately.

Clean Cuts

Not only are these egg wraps portable, they're convenient, too. Make them the night before, wrap them in plastic wrap, and refrigerate. In the morning, pop them into the microwave for a quick breakfast.

Mini Zucchini Pies

Zucchini, cheese, and basil naturally partner with eggs in this Italian-inspired dish. Make it during the summer when zucchini is plentiful to get peak flavor and low price.

¾ cup low-fat (1 percent) milk

1 large egg

3 large egg whites

1 TB. canola oil

1 cup white whole wheat flour or whole wheat flour

1 tsp. baking powder

1 tsp. baking soda

⅛ tsp. sea salt

¼ tsp. ground black pepper

1 tsp. grated lemon zest

4 TB. Parmesan cheese

½ cup onion, diced

1 medium zucchini, grated (about 1½ cups)

2 garlic cloves, peeled and minced

2 tsp. fresh basil, finely chopped

½ cup low-fat cheddar cheese, grated

Yield: 12 zucchini pies
Prep time: 10 minutes
Cook time: 25 minutes
Serving size: 1 pie
Each serving has:
90 calories
4 g total fat
1 g saturated fat
5 g protein
9 g carbohydrate
2 g sugars
24 mg cholesterol
1 g fiber
163 mg sodium

1. Heat the oven to 350°F. Lightly spray a 12-count muffin pan lined with paper muffin cups with cooking spray.

2. In a medium-size bowl, beat milk, eggs, and oil together until well blended. Add flour, baking powder, baking soda, salt, and pepper. Mix well. Stir in lemon zest, Parmesan cheese, onion, zucchini, garlic, and basil.

3. Fill each muffin cup two-thirds full with zucchini mixture. Sprinkle each mini pie with cheddar cheese. Bake for about 25 minutes, until lightly brown and eggs are set.

Variation: This recipe lends itself to any number of variations. Keep the zucchini but you can change the cheese or herb. For instance, swap out the basil for parsley and change the Parmesan to low-fat cheddar or Swiss cheese.

Wholesome Habits

Although most people equate basil with Italian food, it's actually native to India, Asia, and Africa. Its botanical name is *Ocimum basiliscum,* and there are more than 60 varieties. Basil is an aromatic plant in the mint family and is a close cousin to rosemary and thyme.

Baked Spinach-Mushroom Frittata

This fluffy oven-baked frittata uses spinach and mushrooms to keep it moist. Fresh tomatoes and marjoram finish it off in style.

Yield: 1 (16-ounce) casserole
Prep time: 10 minutes
Cook time: 10 to 12 minutes
Serving size: 1 frittata
Each serving has:
231 calories
7 g total fat
2 g saturated fat
18 g protein
25 g carbohydrate
3 g sugars
215 mg cholesterol
4 g fiber
422 mg sodium

½ tsp. garlic, peeled and minced (1 small clove)

1 TB. onion, chopped

½ cup white mushrooms, coarsely chopped

1 cup fresh spinach, chopped

1 large egg

1 large egg white

2 tsp. water

Dash of ground black pepper

2 tsp. spelt flour

½ tsp. baking powder

2 TB. fresh tomato, diced

1 tsp. fresh marjoram leaves, finely chopped

1 TB. low-fat Swiss cheese, grated

1. Heat oven to 425°F. Lightly spray a ceramic 16-ounce casserole dish with cooking spray.

2. Coat a small sauté pan with cooking spray and heat over medium heat. Sauté garlic, onion, mushrooms, and spinach for about 4 minutes until soft. Put in casserole dish and set aside.

3. In a small bowl, mix eggs, water, pepper, flour, and baking powder. Pour egg mixture over spinach. Sprinkle with tomatoes, marjoram, and cheese (in that order). Bake for 10 to 12 minutes until puffed and brown.

Dirty Secrets

Farmers' markets are often great sources for fresh local spinach, but you need to make sure you clean the spinach thoroughly before cooking with it. Spinach grows in loose sandy soil, and its leaves easily trap dirt, sand, grit, and stones. To clean spinach, remove any bruised or damaged leaves and put the leaves in a sink full of cold water. Swirl them around for a few seconds, then let them soak for several minutes. The dirt will sink to the bottom while the leaves float on top.

Mini Mexican Breakfast Pizzas

Who says you can't have pizza for breakfast? Topped with salsa, spinach, and cheese, then baked with a whole egg, this hearty pizza is the perfect eye-opener.

1 batch of Whole Wheat Pizza Dough (see recipe in Chapter 17)

6 TB. low-sodium, all-natural salsa

6 oz. fresh spinach leaves

2 TB. part-skim mozzarella cheese, shredded

6 medium eggs

2 TB. Parmesan cheese

¼ tsp. ground black pepper

Yield: 6 mini pizzas
Prep time: 15 minutes
Cook time: 15 minutes
Serving size: 1 pizza
Each serving has:
429 calories
14 g total fat
3 g saturated fat
18 g protein
61 g carbohydrate
6 g sugars
191 mg cholesterol
10 g fiber
465 mg sodium

1. Heat oven to 450°F. Divide pizza dough into six equal amounts and roll or stretch each one into a 6-inch diameter crust. Fold edges up slightly to form a barrier. Arrange dough on pizza stone or cookie sheet.

2. Heat a small sauté pan, lightly coat with cooking spray, and cook spinach until wilted, about 1 or 2 minutes. Set aside.

3. Spread each pizza with 2 tablespoons of salsa, 1 ounce of spinach, and 1 teaspoon of mozzarella cheese. Bake for 4 minutes. Remove from oven.

4. Using the back of a spoon, gently spread sauce and cheese to outer edge of each pizza, forming an indentation in the dough. Gently break cracked egg into the center of each pizza. Sprinkle each egg with 1 teaspoon of Parmesan cheese and ground black pepper. Bake another 8 to 10 minutes until crust is brown and egg is set.

Wholesome Habits

Unlike American pizzas, which are usually loaded with cheese and meat, pizzas in Italy are traditionally served as individual pies with a smattering of high-quality sauce and cheese and a healthy dose of vegetables.

Chapter 8

Muffins, Breads, and Pancakes

In This Chapter

- ◆ Create delicious healthy breads and muffins
- ◆ Discover the wonderful world of whole grains
- ◆ Prepare pancakes with panache

Store-bought muffins and quick breads are usually loaded with sugar and calories, not to mention a slew of highly processed additives, preservatives, and chemical ingredients. The best way to ensure your baked goods are healthy, clean, and low in fat is to make your own.

Taste and price are also good reasons for opting for home-baked goodies. Although masked by fat and sweeteners, many convenience food muffins and breads can't hide their artificial flavors. And one serving often costs more than what it takes to make an entire loaf of bread or a dozen muffins.

Healthy quick breads are a bit more temperamental than processed ones. Since they are lower in fat and sugar (two ingredients that preserve foods as well as provide flavor) and don't contain any preservatives, their shelf life is shorter than the store-bought variety. So if you don't eat them all in a day or two, your best bet is to freeze the extras.

Creativity Uncovered

The best thing about making your own muffins, breads, and pancakes is that it gives you a tremendous amount of flexibility. You can stick to the basics—like Mom's Favorite Banana Bread or Wild Blueberry Muffins—or get a little creative with options such as Zucchini-Carrot Bread or Pumpkin Oatmeal Pancakes. With home-baked breads, you can tailor your creations to fit your own personal likes and dislikes.

If you do like to experiment, I suggest you expand your horizons with recipes such as Orange Buckwheat Pancakes, Applesauce Walnut Muffins, or Whole Grain Cinnamon Raisin Bread—all found in this chapter. They're worth the effort.

Whole Grain Opportunities

Another advantage of making your own baked goods is upping your fiber intake. Since you won't be using highly processed white flour, whole grain flours become a baking mainstay; fortunately, there is a wide variety of whole grain flours to choose from.

Many of the recipes in this chapter call for small amounts of two flours you may not be familiar with: spelt flour and flaxseed flour, sometimes called flaxseed meal or ground flaxseed. These flours are highly nutritious and packed with fiber, vitamins, and minerals, but they serve an important culinary purpose as well. Spelt flour acts like all-purpose white flour and helps build structure so breads can rise, while flaxseed replaces fat.

Baking may take practice to master, but once you get the hang of it, making homemade baked goodies is easier than you think. And few things are more rewarding than eating a muffin or slice of bread that's still warm from the oven.

Wild Blueberry Muffins

Sweet, wild blueberries pair beautifully with maple syrup and cinnamon. The banana provides sweetness but doesn't overpower the other ingredients.

2 medium bananas, mashed

½ cup unsweetened soymilk

½ cup maple syrup

¼ cup olive oil

1 large egg

1 tsp. vanilla extract

1¾ cups whole wheat pastry flour

½ cup stone-ground cornmeal

1 TB. baking powder

½ tsp. kosher salt

½ tsp. ground cinnamon

1 cup wild blueberries, frozen (not thawed)

Yield: 1 dozen muffins
Prep time: 15 minutes
Cook time: 20 minutes
Serving size: 1 muffin
Each serving has:
184 calories
6 g total fat
1 g saturated fat
4 g protein
32 g carbohydrate
11 g sugars
18 mg cholesterol
3 g fiber
231 mg sodium

1. Preheat the oven to 400°F. Line a 12-cup muffin tin with paper liners, and lightly spray each with cooking spray.

2. In a large bowl, whisk bananas with soymilk, maple syrup, olive oil, egg, and vanilla extract.

3. In a medium bowl, mix together whole wheat pastry flour, cornmeal, baking powder, salt, and cinnamon.

4. Add flour mixture to banana mixture, and stir to combine. Gently fold in frozen blueberries.

5. Spoon mixture into prepared muffin cups, filling each about ¾ full. Bake for 20 minutes or until muffin springs back to the touch. Cool on wire racks.

Variation: For a vegan alternative, omit the egg and decrease the whole wheat pastry flour by ¼ cup.

Wholesome Habits

One of only three berries native to North America, wild blueberries are smaller and more intensely sweet tasting than regular domestic blueberries. They grow best in cool climates and are cultivated in Maine and Canada during six weeks of August and early September. Since they are highly perishable, it's rare to find fresh wild blueberries, but frozen blueberries are available year round in most stores.

Applesauce Walnut Muffins

Combining applesauce and fresh apples is the key to creating this wholesome muffin. Walnuts provide the nutty crunch.

Yield: 12 servings
Prep time: 20 minutes
Cook time: 25 minutes
Serving size: 1 muffin
Each serving has:
236 calories
11 g total fat
2 g saturated fat
4 g protein
32 g carbohydrate
14 g sugars
0 mg cholesterol
3 g fiber
112 mg sodium

½ cup finely chopped fresh apple (about 1 medium apple peeled and cored)

½ cup unsweetened apple-sauce

1 large egg white

½ cup canola oil

½ cup honey

1 tsp. vanilla extract

2 TB. orange juice

1¾ cup whole wheat flour

¾ cup whole wheat pastry flour

¼ tsp. kosher salt

½ tsp. baking soda

½ tsp. baking powder

⅛ tsp. ground cloves

¼ tsp. ground nutmeg

1 tsp. ground cinnamon

¼ cup finely chopped walnuts

1. Preheat the oven to 325°F. Line a 12-cup muffin tin with paper liners, and lightly spray each with cooking spray.

2. In a large bowl, mix apple, applesauce, egg white, canola oil, honey, vanilla, and orange juice.

3. In a medium bowl, whisk together whole wheat flour, whole wheat pastry flour, salt, baking soda, baking powder, and cloves, nutmeg, and cinnamon.

4. Add dry ingredients all at once to wet mixture and stir to combine. Gently mix in chopped walnuts.

5. Spoon mixture into prepared muffin tin, filling each muffin cup about ¾ full. Bake for 25 minutes or until muffin springs back to the touch. Cool on wire racks.

Variation: For an interesting twist, try substituting the same amount of Peach Maple Jam (recipe in Chapter 11) for the applesauce, peeled and pitted peaches for the apple, and maple syrup for the honey.

Clean Cuts

Whole wheat pastry flour is made from soft wheat berries and is a fine, light-colored flour. It's lower in protein than whole wheat flour and so contains less gluten, the protein which gives bread its structure. Use it when you're looking for a tender, lighter, cakelike crumb, but beware that too much can make your bread crumbly and dry.

Mom's Favorite Banana Bread

Enjoy this hearty cinnamon-scented banana bread any time of day—breakfast, lunch, or dinner. The mini chocolate chips satisfy a sweet tooth, but it can work just as well without them.

3 medium bananas, mashed

½ cup canola oil

¼ cup honey

2 tsp. vanilla extract

1 cup whole wheat pastry flour

1 cup whole wheat flour

½ tsp. kosher salt

1 tsp. baking soda

1 tsp. ground cinnamon

2 TB. ground flaxseed

2 large egg whites

2 TB. *Sucanat*

⅓ cup mini chocolate chips

Yield: 1 loaf, 16 servings
Prep time: 25 minutes
Cook time: 30 minutes
Serving size: ¹/₁₆ piece
Each serving has:
180 calories
9 g total fat
1 g saturated fat
3 g protein
24 g carbohydrate
11 g sugars
0 mg cholesterol
2 g fiber
145 mg sodium

1. Preheat oven to 350° F. Spray a 11×7-inch glass pan or 8×8-inch square metal pan with cooking spray.

2. In medium bowl mix together mashed banana, canola oil, honey, and vanilla. Set aside.

3. In a large bowl mix together whole wheat pastry flour, whole wheat flour, salt, baking soda, cinnamon, and flaxseed.

4. In a stand-up mixer beat egg whites on high for 2 minutes until light and frothy. Slowly add Sucanat while still beating. Beat for another 2 minutes until stiff peaks form.

5. Gradually add banana mixture to flour mixture and blend well. Stir in chocolate chips and mix well. Gently fold in egg whites. Pour into pan and bake for 30 minutes or until bread springs back to the touch.

Variation: Omit the chocolate chips and replace with any kind of nuts or dried fruit, such as raisins or dates. For a tropical flair, opt for shredded unsweetened coconut.

Clean Meanings _____

The name **Sucanat** comes from the beginnings of the words SUgar CAne NATural. It is made by extracting the juice from sugar cane, then heating and dehydrating the juice. Because it is minimally processed, this grainy, brown sugar is actually less sweet than regular table sugar, containing 13 percent molasses and 87 percent sucrose. Refined table sugar is 99 percent sucrose. Sucanat has a distinct flavor and molasses-like taste. Rapadura is another dehydrated cane juice on the market.

Zucchini-Carrot Bread

Zucchini and carrots keep this bread moist and flavorful, while maple syrup creates a rich, dark color with a distinctive taste.

1 large egg

1 large egg white

½ cup maple syrup

½ cup canola oil

¾ cup Sucanat

2 TB. orange juice

1½ tsp. vanilla extract

2 cups white whole wheat flour

1 cup whole wheat pastry flour

½ cup spelt flour

2 TB. ground flaxseed

½ tsp. kosher salt

1 tsp. baking soda

½ tsp. baking powder

2 medium zucchini, shredded (about 2 cups)

2 large carrots, peeled and shredded (about 2 cups)

Yield: 2 loaves
(12 slices each)
Prep time: 25 minutes
Cook time: 35 minutes
Serving size: 1 slice
Each serving has:
152 calories
5 g total fat
0 g saturated fat
3 g protein
23 g carbohydrate
11 g sugars
9 mg cholesterol
2 g fiber
113 mg sodium

1. Heat oven to 350°F. Spray two 9×5-inch loaf pans with cooking spray.

2. In a large bowl whisk together eggs, maple syrup, canola oil, Sucanat, orange juice, and vanilla.

3. In a medium bowl mix together whole wheat flour, whole wheat pastry flour, spelt flour, ground flaxseed, salt, baking soda, and baking powder. Dough will be stiff. Stir in shredded zucchini and carrots.

4. Divide batter evenly between two loaf pans and bake for 35 minutes or until toothpick inserted in center comes out clean.

Clean Cuts

Orange juice counteracts the bitterness some people taste in whole wheat breads. All you need is a tablespoon or two to make a difference.

Whole Grain Cinnamon Raisin Bread

Sweet potato is the secret ingredient in this multigrain bread prepared with whole wheat, oatmeal, flaxseed, and spelt. Sweet raisins and a swirl of cinnamon date sugar make it ideal for breakfast, served plain or lightly toasted.

---

*Yield: 2 loaves
(10 slices each loaf)*

Prep time: 15 minutes plus 2 hours rising time

Cook time: 35 to 40 minutes

Serving size: 1 slice

Each serving has:

161 calories

4 g total fat

1 g saturated fat

4 g protein

26 g carbohydrate

8 g sugars

2 mg cholesterol

4 g fiber

76 mg sodium

2½ tsp. active dry yeast (1 package is about 2¼ tsp.)

1 cup warm water (100–110°F)

2 TB. agave nectar or 3 TB. honey

½ cup low-fat (1 percent) milk, warmed in microwave about 30 to 45 seconds

1 medium cooked sweet potato, peeled and mashed (about 1 cup)

3 TB. canola oil

2 TB. orange juice

¾ cup quick cooking dry oatmeal

3 to 4 cups whole wheat flour (for a lighter loaf use 2 cups white whole wheat flour and 1 to 2 cups whole wheat flour)

½ cup spelt flour

½ cup ground flaxseed

½ tsp. sea salt

2 tsp. cinnamon

½ cup date sugar

½ cup raisins

1 TB. unsalted butter, melted

1. In a large bowl, combine yeast, water, and agave nectar. Let sit for 5 minutes until yeast begins to bubble.

2. Add warm milk, sweet potato, canola oil, orange juice, and oatmeal. Mix and let sit for another 5 to 10 minutes to allow oatmeal to soak up liquid.

3. In a small bowl mix 2 cups of whole wheat flour, spelt, flaxseed, and salt. Add all at once to liquid ingredients. Mix until a soft dough forms, adding remaining 1 to 2 cups flour as needed.

4. Knead dough on a floured board or table for 5 to 10 minutes until smooth and elastic. Dough will be slightly sticky.

5. Place dough in large bowl sprayed with cooking spray, cover, and set in a warm place to rise for 1 hour or until nearly doubled in size.

6. Mix cinnamon and date sugar in a small bowl and set aside.

7. Punch down dough. Knead raisins into dough. Divide in half. Spray two 9×5-inch loaf pans with cooking spray (if using stoneware you don't need to spray).

8. Using a rolling pin, roll one half of dough until it's about 8½ inches wide and 12 to 15 inches long, and about ½-inch thick. Brush with ¼ of the melted butter and sprinkle with half the cinnamon-date sugar mixture. Tightly roll from the narrow end, in jellyroll style. Place in loaf pan seam side down. Brush top with melted butter. Repeat step 8 for the other half of dough.

9. Cover with clean dishtowel and let rise until puffed about 1 hour. Heat oven to 375°F. Bake 35 to 40 minutes or until bread is brown and sounds hollow when tapped.

Variation: For whole grain rolls, replace the mashed sweet potato with 1 cup mashed white potato; increase the agave to 3 tablespoons; and omit the raisins, date sugar, and cinnamon. Skip steps 7 and 8. Instead punch down dough and shape into 15 dinner rolls. Place on a cookie sheet sprayed with cooking spray or a baking stone. Cover with clean dishtowel and let rolls rise for 1 hour in a warm place. Bake at 400°F for 25 to 30 minutes. These freeze well.

Clean Cuts

If your raisins are dry, hard, and shriveled, plump them up by soaking them in warm or hot water for 10 to 15 minutes. Drain and pat them dry before using.

Pumpkin Oatmeal Pancakes

Hearty pumpkin is a natural partner for these whole wheat oatmeal pancakes, which are spiced with nutmeg and cinnamon. The finishing touch is a spread of maple applesauce laced with ginger.

Yield: 8 servings (24 pancakes)
Prep time: 10 minutes
Cook time: 15 minutes
Serving size: 3 pancakes
Each serving has:
194 calories
3 g total fat
1 g saturated fat
8 g protein
34 g carbohydrate
12 g sugars
30 mg cholesterol
4 g fiber
442 mg sodium

1 cup quick cooking dry oatmeal

1 cup white whole wheat flour

½ cup whole wheat pastry flour

1 TB. Sucanat

¼ tsp. kosher salt

1 TB. baking powder

1 tsp. baking soda

⅛ tsp. ground nutmeg

¼ tsp. ground cinnamon

1 tsp. olive oil

1 large egg

2 cups low-fat (1 percent) milk

½ cup nonfat, plain Greek yogurt

2 tsp. orange juice

½ cup canned pumpkin

8 tsp. maple syrup

½ cup unsweetened applesauce or Homemade Applesauce (see recipe in Chapter 11)

⅛ tsp. ground ginger

1. Heat a pancake griddle to 300°F.

2. In a medium-size bowl, mix oatmeal, white whole wheat flour, whole wheat pastry flour, Sucanat, salt, baking powder, baking soda, nutmeg, and cinnamon until well blended.

3. In a small bowl, whisk together olive oil, egg, milk, yogurt, orange juice, and pumpkin. Pour into oatmeal mixture and stir just until mixed.

4. Spray hot griddle with cooking spray. Pour batter one spoonful at a time onto hot griddle. Each pancake should be about 4 inches in diameter. Cook slowly until pancake edges are slightly dry and bubbles appear on top, 3 to 4 minutes. Flip and cook another 3 minutes on other side.

5. While pancakes are cooking, mix together maple syrup, applesauce, and ginger in a small bowl.

6. Serve pancakes hot with 1 tablespoon of ginger applesauce maple spread per serving.

Wholesome Habits _____

Canned pumpkin is actually more nutrient dense than fresh pumpkin, mostly because the canned variety has less water in it. Plus most canned pumpkin doesn't have any added salt, sugar, additives, or preservatives. One half-cup serving is only 40 calories, yet it supplies about 300 percent of the recommended dietary allowance (RDA) for vitamin A in the form of beta-carotene. It's also packed with fiber, lutein (good for eyes), and potassium.

Orange Buckwheat Pancakes

Nutty buckwheat combines with orange in this wholesome pancake. Top it with fresh orange sections laced with sweet honey and cinnamon for a special occasion. It's a nice treat to serve when company's over.

Yield: 8 servings *(16 pancakes)*
Prep time: 10 minutes
Cook time: 15 minutes
Serving size: 2 pancakes
Each serving has:
133 calories
2 g total fat
1 g saturated fat
6 g protein
22 g carbohydrate
4 g sugars
28 mg cholesterol
3 g fiber
334 mg sodium

¾ **cup whole grain** *buckwheat* **flour**

1 cup white whole wheat flour

2 tsp. baking powder

1 tsp. baking soda

¼ **tsp. kosher salt**

1 TB. orange juice

1 tsp. orange zest

1 large egg

1 TB. agave nectar

1 cup low-fat or nonfat buttermilk

1 cup unsweetened soymilk

1 tsp. canola oil

1. Heat pancake griddle to 300°F.

2. In a medium bowl, mix together buckwheat flour, white whole wheat flour, baking powder, baking soda, and salt until well blended.

3. In a small bowl, whisk together orange juice, orange zest, egg, agave, buttermilk, soymilk, and oil. Pour into flour mixture and stir just until mixed.

4. Spray hot griddle with cooking spray, then pour batter one spoonful at a time. Each pancake should be about 5 inches in diameter. Cook slowly until pancake edges are slightly dry and bubbles appear on top, 3 to 4 minutes. Flip and cook another 3 minutes on other side.

5. Let pancakes sit for 1 minute before serving. Serve with Honeyed Oranges (see recipe in Chapter 11) or a dollop of yogurt sweetened with vanilla and fresh fruit.

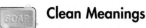 **Clean Meanings**

Buckwheat isn't really a type of wheat at all. In fact, unlike wheat, which is a grass, buckwheat is related to the sorrel and rhubarb family. Although it cooks up like a grain, the kernel is actually the fruit seed. It has a strong distinctive flavor often described as nutty or earthy.

Part 3

Light Bites

Americans love to snack, and it shows—especially around our waists! That's because most snack foods are highly processed fatty foods that are very high in calories. But not the snacks in this book!

In Part 3, you'll find snack recipes that are low in fat and calories and high in flavor. Some of our favorites—Almond Butter Roll-Ups and Clean Deviled Eggs—are substantial enough to be a mini meal, while others—like Date Nut Crisps or Fancy Cheese and Crackers—are just enough to tide you over to the next meal. Then there's our awesome collection of creative fruit-based sauces, salads, salsas, and relishes.

Finally, people who like to drink their snacks rather than eat them will find some wonderful thirst-quenching beverages, such as Carrot Cake Cooler, Cherry Lemonade, and Cranberry Apple Tea. Prepare to be enlightened.

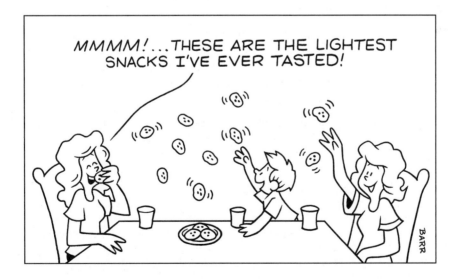

Chapter 9

Mini Munchies

In This Chapter

♦ Snacking on nuts and seeds

♦ Fast 'n' fruity recipes

♦ Planning portable munchies

Since you'll be eating five to six times a day on a clean diet, planning your snacks is just as important as planning your main meals. In fact, you should think of your snacks as mini meals, making sure you include a good balance of nutrients in each one.

All of the snacks in this chapter provide the proper combination of nutrients from a variety of foods. Nuts and seeds top our snack list, and you'll see them throughout this chapter. They're a good source of protein, vitamins, and minerals and have plenty of fiber. Plus, when it comes to nuts and seeds, a little goes a long way. That's important because nuts and seeds are high in fat (good fat, but fat, nonetheless). Often they're paired with fruits like apples, bananas, dates, or raisins. In addition to making a great taste combo, fruits and nuts are a perfect match nutritionally. High-carbohydrate fruits offset the high-fat content of nuts and help keep you going throughout the day.

Another great benefit of nuts, seeds, and nut butters is that they're portable. You can easily bring them with you wherever you go.

Eggs and cheese also make great snacks. Like nuts and seeds, they're nutrient dense (they also supply a concentrated amount of calories, so beware of how much you eat). They do need refrigeration, though, so you might think about investing in a small cooler to keep in your car or at the office. You'll be glad you did.

Pecan Granola

Oats, pecans, and sesame seeds are the basis for this simple granola sweetened with maple syrup. It's great on its own or you can sprinkle it on fruit or yogurt for a sweet pick-me-up.

2 cups quick cooking dry oatmeal	**2 TB. agave nectar**
	2 TB. canola oil
½ cup chopped pecans	**⅓ cup maple syrup**
1 TB. sesame seeds	**Pinch sea salt**

Yield: 10 servings
(about 2 ½ cups)
Prep time: 10 minutes
Cook time: 40 minutes
Serving size: ¼ cup
Each serving has:
169 calories
8 g total fat
1 g saturated fat
3 g protein
23 g carbohydrate
10 g sugars
0 mg cholesterol
2 g fiber
14 mg sodium

1. Preheat the oven to 300°F. In a large bowl, mix oatmeal, pecans, sesame seeds, agave, oil, maple syrup, and salt until combined.

2. Transfer to a cookie sheet and spread evenly into a single layer.

3. Bake 15 minutes then stir with a spatula. Bake another 15 minutes, then stir again and bake another 10 minutes until lightly brown. Remove from oven.

4. Let cool completely then store in an airtight container in a cool place. Granola will keep for 2 to 3 weeks.

Variation: If you like your granola chewier and chunkier, substitute rolled old-fashioned oats for the quick cooking kind, keep your pecans whole, and stir only once, watching carefully and rotating tray to avoid burning. Another option is to switch the nuts for almonds, walnuts, or cashews.

Wholesome Habits

Despite their fat content, a daily handful of pecans can actually reduce your risk of heart disease. One study showed that when added to a healthy diet, pecans lowered bad LDL cholesterol by more than 16 percent and total cholesterol dropped 11 percent compared to diets without pecans. What is it about pecans that makes them so great? High levels of vitamin E and potent phytochemicals.

Trail Mix

This colorful trail mix is loaded with nutritious sunflower and pumpkin seeds. Dried cranberries add a splash of color and tangy sweetness.

Yield: 12 servings
(about 3 cups)
Prep time: 10 minutes
Serving size: ¼ cup
Each serving has:
195 calories
11 g total fat
2 g saturated fat
9 g protein
18 g carbohydrate
8 g sugars
0 mg cholesterol
4 g fiber
47 mg sodium

1 cup dried cranberries, coarsely chopped

½ cup sunflower seeds, unsalted

½ cup roasted pumpkin seeds, salted

1 cup roasted soy nuts, salted

¾ cup roasted peanuts unsalted, shelled

1. In a large bowl mix cranberries, sunflower seeds, pumpkin seeds, soy nuts, and peanuts.

2. Transfer to an airtight container and store for up to three weeks.

Wholesome Habits

George Washington Carver is often credited as the founding father of the peanut industry in the South. During the early 1900s he discovered 300 uses for the legume and promoted the peanut's nutritional and agricultural value, transforming it from a small regional crop to a national commodity. Today we eat more than 6 pounds per capita of peanuts and peanut products annually.

Clean Deviled Eggs

Yogurt gives these deviled eggs their creaminess, while a dash of hot sauce and fresh parsley provide flavorful heat. These eggs are a perfect snack served any time of day.

6 large eggs

1 TB. chopped fresh parsley

½ tsp. hot sauce

⅛ tsp. ground black pepper

½ tsp. yellow prepared mustard

½ tsp. apple cider vinegar or white vinegar

1 TB. low-fat sour cream

2 TB. low-fat plain Greek yogurt

⅛ tsp. garlic powder

Pinch sea salt

Pinch paprika

Yield: 6 servings
Prep time: 10 minutes
Cook time: 12 minutes
Serving size: 2 deviled egg halves
Each serving has:
84 calories
6 g total fat
2 g saturated fat
7 g protein
1 g carbohydrate
1 g sugars
213 mg cholesterol
0 g fiber
80 mg sodium

1. Fill a 2-quart pot with water (about 1 quart) and heat over medium-high heat until water begins to slowly boil. Place one unshelled egg at a time on a spoon and gently lower into water. Eggs should be completely covered with water. Lower temperature to a simmer and cook for 12 minutes.

2. Remove eggs from hot water and transfer to a large bowl filled with cold ice water (make sure eggs are completely covered with water). Let sit until cool enough to handle (about 10 minutes). Peel eggs and cut in half lengthwise. Gently remove egg yolks with a spoon, being careful not to damage egg white. Set egg whites aside.

3. In a small bowl mix egg yolks, parsley, hot sauce, black pepper, mustard, vinegar, sour cream, yogurt, garlic powder, and salt until smooth and creamy.

4. Carefully place a spoonful of yolk mixture into each egg white. Sprinkle with paprika. Serve immediately or refrigerate until ready to serve.

Dirty Secrets

Ever wonder why some boiled egg yolks have a greenish-grey tinge around them? It's because they're overcooked. The best way to avoid this nasty color is to avoid cooking your eggs for too long and to immerse them in ice water as soon as they're done.

Fancy Cheese on Crackers

A far cry from your typical cheese and crackers, this version uses tangy goat cheese, or *chèvre*, to give it some kick and sweet peach maple jam to finish it off. It's a flavor combination you won't soon forget.

Yield: *2 servings*
Prep time: 5 minutes
Serving size: 2 crackers
Each serving has:
174 calories
7 g total fat
4 g saturated fat
6 g protein
22 g carbohydrate
5 g sugars
19 mg cholesterol
4 g fiber
191 mg sodium

1 oz. soft goat cheese

1 oz. low-fat cream cheese

⅛ tsp. grated fresh ginger

4 tsp. Peach Maple Jam (see recipe in Chapter 11) or all-natural fruit-sweetened apricot or peach preserves

Dash cinnamon

4 rye or whole wheat crispbread crackers

4 tsp. sliced almonds

4 medium fresh strawberries, sliced

1. In a small bowl, mix goat cheese and cream cheese until smooth. Add ginger, peach maple jam, and cinnamon. Beat until light and fluffy.

2. Spread one tablespoon of the cheese mixture on top of each crispbread cracker. Top with almonds and strawberry slices. Enjoy.

Clean Meanings

Chèvre (pronounced SHEV-ruh) is the French word for goat and goat cheese. In the United States you will often see goat cheese, imported or not, simply labeled chèvre.

Apples and Nuts

Sometimes the simplest creations are the most sublime. This is one of them—apples and walnuts tossed with orange juice and cinnamon. This is an ideal snack in the fall when apples are plentiful.

2 large apples, skin on, cored, and cut into ½-inch pieces

¼ cup chopped walnuts, toasted

¼ cup orange juice

½ tsp. ground cinnamon

Yield: 3 servings
Prep time: 10 minutes
Serving size: 1 cup
Each serving has:
151 calories
7 g total fat
1 g saturated fat
2 g protein
24 g carbohydrate
16 g sugars
0 mg cholesterol
4 g fiber
2 mg sodium

1. In a large bowl, combine apples, walnuts, orange juice, and cinnamon.

2. Refrigerate until ready to serve.

Variation: This recipe is extremely versatile. Vary the spice by adding ginger, cardamom, cloves, or nutmeg. Vary the nuts by using pecans, almonds, or any type of seed such as pumpkin or sunflower seed. You can even add raisins or other dried fruit, but keep in mind that this will bump up the amount of sugar in your snack.

Clean Cuts

In this recipe, orange juice does more than just add flavor. The ascorbic acid (vitamin C) in it prevents the apples from turning brown. This means you can prepare the apples the night before and they'll still be crisp and white in the morning.

Banana Almond Roll Ups

Banana and peanut butter combine to make a classic comfort food. Here we add a twist by substituting almond butter for peanut butter and increase the fiber by wrapping it in a whole wheat tortilla. A sprinkle of dark chocolate is the icing on the cake.

Yield: 1 serving
Prep time: 5 minutes
Serving size: 1 tortilla
Each serving has:
272 calories
2 g total fat
2 g saturated fat
7 g protein
43 g carbohydrate
11 g sugars
0 mg cholesterol
5 g fiber
342 mg sodium

1 (8-inch) whole wheat tortilla

½ medium banana sliced lengthwise

2 tsp. unsalted, creamy almond butter

1 tsp. dark chocolate (70 to 85 percent dark cacao solids), shaved

1. To assemble, place tortilla on a large flat cutting board or work surface. Lay banana slices in a single layer lengthwise on the bottom middle portion of the tortilla.

2. Spread almond butter on top of banana. Sprinkle with dark chocolate.

3. Fold about 2 inches of the bottom edge of tortilla up towards the center, then fold in each side, one overlapping the other, to enclose banana, and then finish rolling up tortilla. Serve immediately or wrap tightly in plastic wrap and place in an airtight container. Stored in refrigerator, wrap will keep for two to three days.

Variation: If you just can't imagine bananas without peanut butter, skip the almond butter and replace it with all-natural, unsalted peanut butter. Another option is to omit the chocolate and drizzle a small amount of honey instead.

Clean Cuts _____

Nut butters are sold in natural food stores, but they are relatively expensive. Make your own by spreading nuts on a baking sheet and toasting in a 400°F oven for 5 minutes. Then remove any skins and process in a food processor for 2 to 3 minutes. As a general guide the ratio is 2 to 1, so for every 1 cup of nuts you'll get ½ cup butter. The higher the fat content, the creamier the butter.

Date Coconut Crisps

These chewy *dates* are coated with coconut and oatmeal, but the best part is the hidden surprise inside—a whole almond.

18 whole, pitted dates (California variety)

18 whole almonds

1½ tsp. *arrowroot*

1 fresh egg white

4 tsp. unsweetened, shredded coconut

¼ cup quick cooking dry oatmeal

Yield: 6 servings		
Prep time: 10 minutes		
Cook time: 7 minutes		
Serving size: 3 dates		
Each serving has:		
107 calories		
3 g total fat		
1 g saturated fat		
2 g protein		
20 g carbohydrate		
13 g sugars		
0 mg cholesterol		
2 g fiber		
11 mg sodium		

1. Heat oven to 400°F. Push one almond into the center of each date.

2. Place arrowroot in a plastic bag along with dates. Seal and shake until dates are well-coated.

3. Beat egg white in a small bowl. Place coated dates in the bowl with egg white. Gently toss to cover.

4. In a second plastic bag add coconut and oatmeal. Transfer coated dates to second bag, seal, and shake gently until all dates are coated with coconut mixture.

5. Place dates on cookie sheet or baking stone and bake for 6 to 7 minutes or until lightly brown. Remove from oven and let cool. Serve when warm or refrigerate. Dates will keep about a week in the refrigerator. They also freeze well.

Clean Meanings

Dates are a sturdy fruit popular in Middle Eastern and Mediterranean cuisines. They are a good source of fiber and potassium as well as sugar.

Arrowroot is a white powder ground from the root of a West Indian plant. It looks similar to cornstarch (because it's highly refined, cornstarch is not included on the clean diet) and is used as a thickener in most culinary applications.

Chapter 10

Delicious Dips and Spreads

In This Chapter

◆ Lean, low-calorie classics

◆ Easy Mediterranean-inspired must-haves

◆ Lightening up sweet, creamy dessert dips

Dips and spreads make great snacks, especially if you pair them with crackers, raw vegetables, a hard-boiled egg, or fruits.

Plus, they are super simple to make. Most only use a few ingredients, which you can throw right into the food processor, then just whiz away. Dips and spreads are also portable and convenient. Prepare them the night before and pack them away for the next day's breakfast or lunch. Keep them in a cooler in your car and bring them to work. You can even make one big batch and eat it all week long.

Making your own dips and spreads will save you money and calories. Store-bought brands are usually laden with fat, salt, and sugar and they can be expensive compared to the pennies it takes to make your own. Homemade versions are also high on flavor, since they don't rely on those dirty ingredients—salt, sugar, and fat—for taste. You'll be certain to notice a difference.

Spinach and Artichoke Dip

Try serving this classic combination of spinach and artichoke mellowed out with cream cheese and cottage cheese the next time you have guests. They won't even know they're eating clean.

Yield: 6 servings
Prep time: 20 minutes
Serving size: ⅓ cup
Each serving has:
61 calories
2 g total fat
1 g saturated fat
5 g protein
6 g carbohydrate
1 g sugars
7 mg cholesterol
3 g fiber
205 mg sodium

1 (10-oz.) package frozen spinach, thawed and squeezed dry

6 oz. frozen artichoke hearts, thawed

2 cloves garlic, peeled and chopped

2 oz. low-fat cream cheese

2 TB. Parmesan cheese, grated

4 TB. low-fat cottage cheese

1 TB. lemon juice

2 TB. green onion, chopped

2 TB. red bell pepper, chopped

1 TB. fresh basil, chopped

¼ tsp. ground black pepper

⅛ tsp. sea salt (optional)

1. Place spinach, artichoke hearts, garlic, cream cheese, Parmesan cheese, cottage cheese, lemon juice, green onion, red pepper, basil, pepper, and salt (if using) in food processor. Process on high speed for about 40 seconds. Stop and scrape down the sides of the bowl with a spatula. Process another 30 or 40 seconds until smooth.

2. Place in serving bowl and set out with crackers, celery, and carrot sticks or baked whole wheat chips.

Clean Cuts

If you want to use fresh spinach instead of frozen, sauté 6 cups of packed fresh spinach in 1 teaspoon of olive oil, along with the garlic and the green onion over medium heat. Cover for 1 or 2 minutes until wilted. Cooking the spinach first, will ensure that your dip isn't watery.

Get Crabby Dip

Crab dips don't have to be loaded with cheese and fatty sour cream to grab your taste buds. Fresh parsley and dill along with lemon zest give this light version its vibrancy.

4 oz. lump crabmeat	**1 tsp. lemon zest**
¼ cup fresh parsley, finely chopped	**⅛ tsp. ground black pepper**
4 sprigs fresh dill or fennel, finely chopped (about 2 tsp.)	**Dash of sea salt (optional)**
	1 oz. low-fat cream cheese
¾ cup cucumber, peeled, seeded, and diced (about ½ medium cucumber)	**2 TB. silken soft tofu**
	2 TB. low-fat sour cream
1 TB. red onion, finely chopped	**½ tsp. lemon juice**
	½ tsp. hot sauce or to taste

> *Yield: 4 servings*
>
> **Prep time:** 15 minutes
> **Serving size:** ¼ cup
>
> **Each serving has:**
> 52 calories
> 2 g total fat
> 1 g saturated fat
> 5 g protein
> 3 g carbohydrate
> 1 g sugars
> 23 mg cholesterol
> 0 g fiber
> 176 mg sodium

1. In a large bowl, gently blend crabmeat with parsley, dill, cucumber, red onion, lemon zest, black pepper, and salt (if using).

2. In a medium bowl, beat cream cheese, tofu, sour cream, lemon juice, and hot sauce until light and fluffy.

3. Gently fold whipped cream cheese mixture into crab mixture all at once. Be careful not to break up crab.

4. Serve immediately plain or with crackers.

Variation: Vary the seafood by replacing the crab with the same amount of fresh cooked tuna or salmon.

Clean Cuts

Double the serving size of this delightful crab dip and place on top of mixed greens or fresh baby spinach for a salad, roll it into a wrap, or spread it on a sandwich.

Spicy Hummus

Puréed chickpeas are the basis behind this Middle Eastern spread seasoned with lemon, garlic, and a shot of hot sauce. Spooned into a pita it also makes a great main meal.

Yield: 8 servings
Prep time: 10 minutes
Serving size: ¼ cup
Each serving has:
135 calories
7 g total fat
1 g saturated fat
6 g protein
14 g carbohydrate
3 g sugars
0 mg cholesterol
3 g fiber
62 mg sodium

2 cups canned chickpeas (14-oz. can), drained and rinsed

2 TB. unsalted, all-natural almond butter

¼ tsp. ground cumin

¼ cup packed parsley sprigs

1 tsp. hot sauce

3 TB. lemon juice

¼ cup nonfat, plain Greek yogurt

2 garlic cloves, peeled and crushed

⅛ tsp. ground black pepper

2 TB. extra-virgin olive oil

1. Place chickpeas, almond butter, cumin, parsley, hot sauce, lemon juice, yogurt, garlic, black pepper, salt, and olive oil in a food processor. Process on high speed. Stop occasionally to scrape down sides. Process until dip is smooth and creamy, approximately 2 to 3 minutes.

2. Taste and add more lemon juice or hot sauce if necessary. Serve at room temperature or chilled.

Variation: Hummus is extremely versatile. You can up the garlic; add roasted red pepper, black olives, or sun-dried tomatoes; or change it up with fresh herbs like basil or cilantro. Give it a kick with different spices, too, like chili powder or curry powder. Let your imagination and your taste buds guide you.

Clean Cuts

This is one case when canned is better than fresh, only because canned chickpeas are precooked and thus softer than fresh, giving the processed hummus a smoother texture. If you do decide to cook from fresh, be sure and cook the chickpeas well, and add about ⅛ teaspoon sea salt.

Tomato *Bruschetta*

Italian food is at its best when it's at its simplest, and nothing could be simpler than this tomato, basil, and garlic topping seasoned with a touch of cheese, lemon, and olive oil served on whole wheat toast.

2 medium tomatoes, seeded and cut into ¼-inch pieces

1 TB. plus 1 tsp. fresh basil, finely chopped

2 TB. fresh parsley, finely chopped

2 garlic cloves, peeled and minced

1 tsp. balsamic vinegar

2 TB. plus 1 tsp. extra-virgin olive oil

1 tsp. lemon zest

1 tsp. grated sharp Italian cheese like Grana Padano, Parmesan, or Pecorino Romano

¼ tsp. ground black pepper

⅛ tsp. sea salt (optional)

4 thick slices multigrain or whole wheat Italian bread

Yield: 4 servings
Prep time: 15 minutes
Serving size: ¼ cup plus 1 slice of whole wheat bread
Each serving has:
196 calories
10 g total fat
2 g saturated fat
6 g protein
21 g carbohydrate
4 g sugars
0 mg cholesterol
4 g fiber
256 mg sodium

1. In a large bowl, mix tomatoes, basil, parsley, garlic, balsamic vinegar, 2 tablespoons olive oil, lemon zest, cheese, black pepper, and salt (if using) until blended.

2. Let rest for 5 to 10 minutes. Toast whole wheat bread in toaster or under broiler. Brush each slice with 1 teaspoon olive oil. Place on flat work surface and cut each slice into four pieces.

3. To assemble, place 1 tablespoon of tomato mixture on top of each piece of whole wheat bread. Serve 4 pieces tomato bruschetta per person.

Clean Meanings _____

Bruschetta (pronounced broo-SKEH-tah) comes from the Italian word *buscare* which means "to roast over coals." In its simplest form, it is thick Tuscan bread toasted and then rubbed with garlic and olive oil. Today we add chopped seasoned tomatoes as a topping, hence the name tomato bruschetta.

Red Pepper and Eggplant Spread

Hot weather vegetables like red pepper and eggplant are staples in Mediterranean countries. Roasted and puréed with garlic and fresh herbs, they taste luxuriously rich with few calories.

Yield: 4 servings
Prep time: 10 minutes
Cook time: 45 minutes
Serving size: ⅓ cup
Each serving has:
86 calories
4 g total fat
1 g saturated fat
2 g protein
13 g carbohydrate
5 g sugars
0 mg cholesterol
6 g fiber
151 mg sodium

1 large eggplant (about 1¼ lb.), cut vertically down the center

1 large sweet red pepper

8 garlic cloves

4 TB. fresh basil, coarsely chopped

4 tsp. fresh marjoram or oregano leaves

¼ tsp. ground black pepper

2 TB. extra-virgin olive oil

¼ tsp. sea salt

2 tsp. lemon juice

1. Heat oven to 425°F. Spray a large 13×9 roasting pan with cooking spray. Then place eggplant halves skin side up, whole red pepper, and garlic cloves (with skin on). Lightly spray vegetables with cooking spray. Roast in oven uncovered for 45 minutes.

2. While vegetables are roasting, place basil, marjoram, black pepper, olive oil, salt, and lemon juice in a food processor with chopping blade. Set aside.

3. When vegetables are done, remove from oven and let cool for 5 minutes. Peel off skin and take out seeds from pepper. Squeeze garlic pulp from cloves into food processor with herbs. Scoop eggplant meat from skin and put into a small bowl. Remove seeds. They will come out in large clusters.

4. Place eggplant and red pepper in food processor with herb and garlic mixture. Process on high speed. Pause every 10 seconds to scrape down sides with a spatula, for a total of 30 seconds. Mixture will be chunky, similar to a salsa.

5. Serve immediately or at room temperature.

Clean Cuts

Salting eggplant before cooking removes any bitterness it might have. The best way to do this is to take raw eggplant slices, sprinkle with coarse salt, and let sit for 30 minutes. Then rinse or wipe salt off, squeeze eggplant dry, and cook.

Creamy Berry Dip

All natural fruit-sweetened jam is the secret behind this sweet creamy dip. Here we've used blueberries, but any kind of berry or sweet fruit—strawberry, blackberry, dark cherry, peach, or apricot—will do.

¼ cup low-fat cottage cheese

4 oz. low-fat cream cheese (¼ cup)

4 TB. all natural, fruit-sweetened blueberry or blackberry spread

2 sprigs fresh mint

Yield: 4 servings
Prep time: 5 minutes
Serving size: ¼ cup
Each serving has:
106 calories
4 g total fat
3 g saturated fat
4 g protein
13 g carbohydrate
9 g sugars
16 mg cholesterol
0 g fiber
189 mg sodium

1. Place cottage cheese, cream cheese, fruit spread, and mint in a food processor. Process on high for about 1 minute. Stop occasionally to scrape down the sides. Process again for another minute until smooth and creamy.

2. Serve with crackers, fresh fruit, or crudité vegetables.

Clean Cuts

All-natural, fruit-sweetened spreads usually have less sugar and fewer calories than regular brands. They are not loaded with refined sugars like high-fructose corn syrup, either.

Peanutty Dip

Lightening up peanut butter and banana with *tofu* is a great way to cut calories without sacrificing taste.

Yield: 8 servings
Prep time: 5 minutes
Serving size: 3 table-spoons
Each serving has:
112 calories
8 g total fat
2 g saturated fat
5 g protein
7 g carbohydrate
3 g sugars
0 mg cholesterol
1 g fiber
3 mg sodium

1 medium ripe banana

½ cup all-natural creamy or crunchy unsalted, peanut butter

3 TB. silken soft tofu

¼ tsp. vanilla extract

1. Mash banana, peanut butter, tofu, and vanilla extract in a small bowl with fork until smooth and creamy. (Or you can place banana, peanut butter, tofu, and vanilla in a food processor. Process on high speed for about 30 seconds, scrape down sides, then process another minute until smooth and creamy.)

2. Serve immediately with crackers, celery sticks, carrot sticks, or strawberries. You can also thinly spread on a whole wheat pita, roll, and slice into pinwheels.

3. To store, press plastic wrap over surface of dip to prevent any air from getting at it and place in a sealed air-tight container. This dip is best eaten the day it's made.

Variation: For a twist, replace the vanilla with orange zest.

 Clean Meanings

Tofu is a mildly-flavored food made from pressed soybeans and formed into a smooth curd. The three most common types are silken soft tofu, which is best blended into creamy soups, dips, or salad dressings; firm or regular tofu, which is an all-purpose tofu used for stir-fries, soups, and mixed dishes; and extra-firm tofu, which is good for grilling, tofu steaks, or kebobs. You can usually find all three varieties in the refrigerator or produce section of the supermarket.

Chapter 11

Fruitful Endeavors

In This Chapter

- Fruity sauces and jams to sweeten your day
- Substantial salsas make a meal
- Cool your taste buds with soothing slaws and chutneys

Now it's time to broaden your palate and expand your culinary prowess with zesty salsas, fruity jams and sauces, and spicy chutneys. Each of the recipes featured in this chapter includes some kind of fresh herb or intriguing spice mixed with flavorful, clean ingredients. The combinations may surprise you, but they are also meant to inspire and excite you.

Pear Ginger Chutney, Peach Maple Jam, Honeyed Oranges—certainly this food is anything but boring! Best of all, dishes like this prove that food doesn't have to be loaded with salt, sugar, and fat to be delicious. Nor does it have to be loaded with calories. Serve these zippy sauces to your family and they will never know they're eating clean.

Flavorful doesn't mean hot, either. Although these recipes are chock full of herbs and spices, most are not spicy hot, though if you like heat, it's easy to adjust the seasonings to suit your taste.

These sauces are also quick and easy to whip up. Some can even be made a day or more ahead of time. Versatility on the plate is another bonus, as they can be served as a side with a protein—like shrimp, chicken, or fish—or as the highlight of the meal on grains or salads. When eaten with whole grain crackers and low-fat cheese, they can also stand in for a snack. (Yes, even the salsas are substantial enough to make a mini meal, and the applesauce is absolutely heavenly all by itself.)

So throw on your apron and start chopping—it's time to impress your taste buds!

Clean Tomato Avocado Corn Salsa

This chunky salsa, which highlights tomato, corn, and avocado, is brightened with a splash of lime and a sprinkle of cilantro. It's so good, you could easily eat it on its own as a small salad.

1 garlic clove, peeled and minced

1 TB. onion, finely chopped

2 TB. fresh cilantro, finely chopped

½ cup corn kernels (about 1 ear of corn), fresh or thawed from frozen

½ small avocado, cut into ¼-inch pieces

½ medium tomato, chopped into ¼-inch pieces

1 tsp. olive oil

1 TB. lime juice

⅛ tsp. coarse black pepper

⅛ tsp. sea salt

Yield: 5 servings
Prep time: 15 minutes
Serving size: ¼ cup
Each serving has:
80 calories
6 g total fat
1 g saturated fat
1 g protein
7 g carbohydrate
1 g sugars
0 mg cholesterol
3 g fiber
62 mg sodium

1. If using fresh corn, shuck corn and place in boiling water for about 8 minutes or until tender. Remove corn from water and let rest until cool enough to handle. Stand on end and carefully cut off kernels with a sharp knife. Measure ½ cup. Save extra corn for another use.

2. In a medium bowl, gently mix garlic, onion, cilantro, corn, avocado, tomato, olive oil, and lime juice. Sprinkle with black pepper and salt, and toss together.

3. Serve with grilled chicken or shrimp, use as topping on whole wheat crackers or crispbreads, or as dressing on a green salad.

Wholesome Habits

Botanically speaking, the tomato is a fruit, not a vegetable. Any juicy, pulpy part of a plant that surrounds the seeds is considered a fruit. However, the U.S. Supreme Court didn't see it that way when, in 1887, they legally declared the tomato a vegetable.

Mango Pineapple Salsa

A take-off on Caribbean flavors, this sweet and spicy *salsa* pairs mango and pineapple with two unlikely spices—hot chili powder and allspice.

Yield: 4 servings
Prep time: 10 minutes
Serving size: ½ cup
Each serving has:
61 calories
0 g total fat
0 g saturated fat
1 g protein
16 g carbohydrate
12 g sugars
0 mg cholesterol
2 g fiber
3 mg sodium

1 mango, peeled, pitted, and cut into ½-inch pieces (about 1 cup)

1 cup fresh pineapple, cut into ¼-inch pieces

3 TB. sweet red pepper, finely diced

1 TB. green onion, chopped

½ tsp. orange zest

2 TB. orange juice

¼ tsp. ground chili powder

⅛ tsp. ground allspice

Cayenne (optional)

1. In a large bowl mix mango, pineapple, red pepper, onion, orange zest, orange juice, chili powder, allspice, and cayenne (if using), together.

2. Serve on its own or as an accompaniment to chicken, fish, or pork. This salsa will also work well with any bean or grain.

 Clean Meanings

Salsa is the Spanish word for "sauce." Most people equate salsa with tomato-based sauces, but you can create countless versions of salsas using many different ingredients besides tomatoes.

Honeyed Oranges

Fresh basil or mint adds a surprising twist to ripe orange chunks, while a drizzle of honey kisses this dish with sweetness. If you like your fruit a little less green, substitute a sprinkle of cinnamon for the fresh chopped herb.

4 medium navel oranges, peeled and white pith removed, cut into pieces (about 2 cups bite-size pieces of orange sections)

4 tsp. honey

1 TB. shredded fresh basil or mint

Yield: 4 servings
Prep time: 15 minutes
Serving size: ½ cup
Each serving has:
67 calories
0 g total fat
0 g saturated fat
1 g protein
17 g carbohydrate
15 g sugars
0 mg cholesterol
2 g fiber
0 mg sodium

1. In a large bowl toss orange pieces, honey, and basil or mint. Let sit at room temperature for 20 minutes so fruit can release juice and absorb flavor.

2. Serve immediately or refrigerate until ready to use.

Variation: To make honeyed orange pancake syrup, (see recipe for Orange Buckwheat Pancakes in Chapter 8) increase the honey to 4 tablespoons and replace the basil with ¼ teaspoon cinnamon. Makes 8 (¼ cup) servings.

Wholesome Habits

Orange varieties number in the dozens and include both sweet and bitter or sour varieties. Among the sweets the best known are navel, a good eating orange; Valencia, the king of juice oranges; and blood oranges, which have a dark red burgundy flesh. The most common sour orange you're likely to see is the Seville from Spain.

Pear Ginger Chutney

The American South has a long tradition of slow-cooking fruits with spices, vinegar, and sugar, which is exactly what *chutney* is. In this rendition, pears and raisins combine with ginger and curry for an Indian twist.

Yield: 8 servings
Prep time: 15 minutes
Cook time: 45 minutes
Serving size: ¼ cup
Each serving has:
85 calories
0 g total fat
0 g saturated fat
1 g protein
22 g carbohydrate
16 g sugars
0 mg cholesterol
2 g fiber
75 mg sodium

2 medium pears, peeled, cored, and diced

¾ cup raisins

½ cup onion, finely chopped

1 tsp. fresh ginger, finely chopped

1 TB. honey

½ tsp. curry powder

¼ tsp. ground black pepper

¼ tsp. sea salt

1 tsp. apple cider vinegar or white vinegar

½ tsp. fresh rosemary leaves, finely chopped (optional)

⅓ cup water

1. In large bowl gently mix pears, raisins, onion, ginger, honey, curry, black pepper, salt, vinegar, and rosemary (if using).

2. Pour fruit mixture into a medium-size pot and place on low heat. Add water, mix, and cover. Cook for 45 minutes, stirring occasionally, until fruit is soft.

3. Let chutney cool. Serve at room temperature or refrigerate until cold, then serve. This chutney tastes even better the next day when the flavors have a chance to blend. The chutney can be stored in an airtight container in the refrigerator for up to 1 week.

Clean Meanings

Chutney is an Indian word, which comes from the Hindi word chatni, which means "for licking." In India chutney is a common condiment made from fresh ingredients and usually very spicy hot. When the English picked it up in the 1600s, they started cooking their chutney into a thick jamlike consistency minus the heat. American versions are similar to the English.

Great Guacamole

Serve this creamy, smooth dip when Mexican food is on the menu. Its bright, lively taste is addictive.

2 medium Hass avocadoes, coarsely chopped

2 drops hot sauce (optional)

2 tsp. low-fat or lite sour cream

2 tsp. green onions, finely chopped (both green and white)

2 oz. silken soft tofu

4 tsp. lime juice

2 tsp. cilantro, chopped

⅛ tsp. cracked black pepper

Yield: 7 *servings*
Prep time: 10 minutes
Serving size: 3 table-spoons
Each serving has:
99 calories
9 g total fat
1 g saturated fat
2 g protein
5 g carbohydrate
1 g sugars
1 mg cholesterol
4 g fiber
6 mg sodium

1. Place avocado, hot sauce (if using), sour cream, green onions, tofu, lime juice, cilantro, and black pepper in a food processor. Process on high speed until smooth, approximately 1 minute. Stop occasionally to scrape down the sides until a smooth consistency has been reached.

2. Serve with crispbreads, baked whole wheat pita chips, or baked corn tortillas. Guacamole also makes an excellent accompaniment to burritos, Mexican pizza, or fajitas.

Clean Cuts

To keep guacamole from turning brown, lay a piece of plastic wrap directly on top of the dip (pressing gently down all around so there are no air pockets). Then cover the bowl with another piece of plastic and refrigerate.

Cucumber Yogurt Slaw

The cooling combination of yogurt and cucumber is kicked up a notch by peppery watercress and spicy cayenne. Serve this Indian-inspired dish as a side, salad, or condiment to meats and grains.

Yield: 3 servings
Prep time: 10 minutes
Serving size: ⅓ cup
Each serving has:
48 calories
0 g total fat
0 g saturated fat
6 g protein
6 g carbohydrate
5 g sugars
0 mg cholesterol
0 g fiber
123 mg sodium

½ *English cucumber* (about a 6-inch long piece), grated

1 TB. fresh fennel or dill leaves, finely chopped

2 tsp. fresh mint, finely chopped

¼ cup watercress, coarsely chopped

6 oz. nonfat, plain Greek yogurt

¼ tsp. ground cumin

1 tsp. honey (optional)

⅛ tsp. cayenne

⅛ tsp. sea salt

1. Squeeze the grated cucumber with your hands to get as much water out as possible. Place in a large bowl.

2. To cucumber add fennel, mint, watercress, yogurt, cumin, honey (if using), cayenne, and sea salt. Mix well with a wooden spoon. Serve immediately with crispbread crackers.

Clean Meanings

English cucumbers are longer and thinner than regular cucumbers. They also have smaller seeds, and fewer of them, so they're not as watery. Since they are not waxed, they're sold wrapped in plastic. In this recipe a regular cucumber will also work; just be sure to peel and seed the cucumber before grating.

Homemade Baked Applesauce

You don't have to toil over a hot stove with this no-fuss recipe. The apples are simply baked with cinnamon and a bit of honey.

3½ lb. apples (about 7 or 8 medium apples), peeled, cored, and roughly sliced (MacIntosh, Gala, Fuji, Cortland, or Pippin are best, but any apple or combination of apples will work)

4 TB. water

1 tsp. ground cinnamon

2 TB. fresh lemon juice squeezed from ½ lemon

2 TB. honey

2 TB. orange juice

1 tsp. vanilla extract

Cayenne (optional)

Yield: 12 servings (4 cups)
Prep time: 30 minutes
Cook time: 1 hour and 15 minutes
Serving size: ⅓ cup
Each serving has:
73 calories
0 g total fat
0 g saturated fat
0 g protein
19 g carbohydrate
15 g sugars
0 mg cholesterol
3 g fiber
1 mg sodium

1. Heat oven to 300°F. In a large bowl mix apples with water, cinnamon, lemon juice, honey, orange juice, and vanilla until evenly coated.

2. Pour into 13×9-inch roasting pan and spread evenly. Cover tightly with aluminum foil. Bake in oven for 45 minutes. Take out of oven, uncover, and stir. Put cover tightly back on and bake for another 45 minutes.

3. When done remove from oven. If using cayenne, sprinkle it in. Let cool for a few minutes. Mash with a potato masher until chunky. You can also place apples in a food processor for a smoother consistency.

4. Serve warm or cold. Place in an airtight container and refrigerate. Applesauce will keep up to 2 weeks.

Clean Cuts

Applesauce freezes beautifully. Make a big batch, divide it up, and you'll have homemade applesauce all year long.

Peach Maple Jam

This peach maple jam isn't like most jams—it's more like a thick peachy sauce with a hint of maple. It's perfect as an accompaniment to pork or chicken.

Yield: 6 servings (1½ cups)
Prep time: 10 minutes
Cook time: 35 minutes
Serving size: ¼ cup
Each serving has:
58 calories
0 g total fat
0 g saturated fat
1 g protein
15 g carbohydrate
13 g sugars
0 mg cholesterol
1 g fiber
1 mg sodium

1 lb. peaches (3–4 large), peeled, pitted, and sliced

½ cup water

1 TB. agave nectar

2 TB. maple syrup

¼ tsp. ground cinnamon

Sea salt

¼ tsp. arrowroot

1. Place peaches and water in a medium saucepan over medium-high heat.

2. Bring to low boil and cook for 10 to 15 minutes until peaches begin to break down. Add agave, maple syrup, cinnamon, and pinch of salt. Cook for another 10 to 15 minutes, until peaches are soft. Add arrowroot and cook another 5 minutes.

3. Let cool. Peaches will thicken upon sitting. Store in an airtight container in refrigerator. Peach sauce will keep 2 weeks. Serve cold or hot.

Variation: When apricots are in season, make an apricot maple jam. Replace peaches with 1 pound pitted and peeled fresh apricots (about 7 apricots).

 Clean Cuts

Cooking up sauces, jams, and chutneys is a great way to use up damaged, bruised, or overripe fruit.

Chapter 12

Thirst Quenchers

In This Chapter

- ◆ Creamy milk-based coolers
- ◆ Fabulously fizzy drinks
- ◆ Antioxidant-rich tasty teas

Just because you've cut out soft drinks and sweetened juices doesn't mean water is your only option. Milk, unsweetened or naturally sweetened 100 percent fruit juice, and teas are clean as long as you watch how much you gulp down.

Unfortunately, most people don't pay attention to the calorie-content of their favorite drinks. High calorie flavored coffee drinks, smoothies, and specialty shakes can easily tack on an extra 400 or 500 calories to your diet—as much as a whole meal!

Worse yet, most of these calories come from simple or highly refined sugars, so they're absorbed quickly, spiking blood glucose levels and packing on the fat. The recipes in this chapter control the sugars as well as the calories. Most have only a touch of sweetness, allowing the true flavor of the juice or tea to shine through.

As a general rule, try to dilute fruit juices with a sugar-free beverage like water, sparkling water, or unsweetened tea. Another tip is to look for juices with 100 percent juice of the fruit named on the front label (look in the ingredient list). Many times pear, grape, and apple juice are used as cheaper fillers, increasing the sweetness of the drink while still allowing it to be called "100 percent juice."

Finally, be creative. Water with a twist of lemon or lime is fine, but think about adding a splash of pineapple, or some sliced strawberries, or perhaps a sprig of spearmint.

Carrot Cake Cooler

This drink tastes like carrot cake in a glass with about half the fat and calories. It's ideal when you want something filling and satisfying.

**6 TB. all-natural unsweet-
ened carrot juice**

**3 TB. reduced-fat (lite)
coconut milk**

**3 TB. unsweetened pineapple
juice**

4 TB. unsweetened soymilk

Cinnamon and nutmeg

1. In a large glass mix carrot juice, coconut milk, pineapple juice, and soymilk. Stir with spoon.

2. Add ice cubes. Sprinkle with cinnamon and nutmeg and serve.

Clean Cuts _____

Although you can make your own carrot juice with a juicer, you can easily find it at natural food stores, usually in the refrigerator section of the produce department or packaged in aseptic packaging on the shelf near the fruit juices. Carrot juice tastes surprisingly sweet and is high in beta-carotene (a form of vitamin A).

Yield: 1 serving
Prep time: 5 minutes
Serving size: 1 cup
Each serving has:
105 calories
3 g total fat
3 g saturated fat
2 g protein
16 g carbohydrate
8 g sugars
0 mg cholesterol
1 g fiber
68 mg sodium

Dark Chocolate Soymilk

Prepare this hot dark chocolate milk on a cold winter night. This rich, creamy drink with cinnamon and vanilla notes is soothing and delicious.

Yield: 1 serving
Prep time: 5 minutes
Serving size: 1 cup
Each serving has:
177 calories
8 g total fat
4 g saturated fat
8 g protein
17 g carbohydrate
5 g sugars
0 mg cholesterol
4 g fiber
157 mg sodium

**1 square (½ oz.) dark choco-
late, with 70 percent or more
cacao solids**

¼ tsp. cocoa powder

1 cup unsweetened soymilk

½ tsp. vanilla extract

1 tsp. black coffee

Cinnamon

1. In a small glass bowl, melt dark chocolate with cocoa powder in the microwave for 30 to 45 seconds, stirring every 10 seconds.

2. Pour soymilk in a glass and microwave until warm, about 1 minute, or heat in small saucepan over medium heat until hot but not boiling.

3. In a small bowl, whisk 2 tablespoons warm soymilk into chocolate, blending thoroughly. While still whisking add ¼ cup more soymilk, and then remaining soymilk. Blend until smooth.

4. Whisk in vanilla, coffee, and a pinch of cinnamon. Pour into a mug and serve hot, or refrigerate and serve cold.

Wholesome Habits _____

Dark chocolate is better for you than white or milk choco-
late, thanks to its health-promoting antioxidants. Although a bit higher in fat than white and milk chocolate, dark chocolate has less sugar and more cocoa. The best ones boast 70 percent or more cacao solids right on the label.

Acai Berry Fizzle

Acai berry has a tart berry taste with hints of chocolate. Here it's combined with sparkling water and a twist of lime for a refreshing drink.

4 oz. acai berry juice

4 oz. sparkling water

1 thin lime wedge

Yield: 1 serving
Prep time: 5 minutes
Serving size: 1 cup
Each serving has:
45 calories
0 g total fat
0 g saturated fat
0 g protein
11 g carbohydrate
8 g sugars
0 mg cholesterol
0 g fiber
0 mg sodium

1. In a tall 10-ounce glass, pour acai berry juice and sparkling water over ice. Stir. Garnish with twist of lime. Serve immediately.

Variation: If you can't find acai berry juice, use 100 percent pomegranate or cranberry juice. Since pomegranate juice is more concentrated and sweeter than acai berry juice, you need less. Replace acai juice with 3 ounces of pomegranate juice and increase the sparkling water to 5 ounces. Pour over ice and serve. Do the same for cranberry juice.

 Clean Meanings

Acai berry comes from the acai palm tree, which is native to the Amazon region of Brazil. Since fresh acai berries are too fragile to travel, they're only available dried, frozen (as a pulp), or in juice form. Because of its strong tart taste, most acai juice is blended with mango, apple, or other sweet fruits. Acai berry is known for its high antioxidant content.

Citrus Blast

Enjoy this citrusy blend of lemon, lime, and orange juice on a hot summer day. It can be made with plain or sparkling water.

Yield: 5 servings
Prep time: 5 minutes
Serving size: 1 cup
Each serving has:
57 calories
0 g total fat
0 g saturated fat
0 g protein
15 g carbohydrate
13 g sugars
0 mg cholesterol
0 g fiber
1 mg sodium

1 qt. plain filtered tap water or sparkling water

Juice from 1 large orange

Zest from 1 large orange (use the same orange from juice), about 2 TB.

Juice from 1 large lemon

Juice from 1 large lime

Zest from 1 lime (use the same lime from juice), about 1 tsp.

3 TB. agave nectar

Fresh mint

1. In a 2-quart pitcher add water, orange juice and zest, lemon juice, lime juice and zest, and agave. Mix with wooden spoon.

2. Pour 8 ounces each over ice into 5 large glasses. Garnish each with a sprig of mint. Serve immediately.

Clean Cuts

Fill an ice cube tray with citrus blast and freeze. Use cubes to chill sparkling water, plain water, or orange juice for a citrusy twist.

Cherry Lemonade

Nothing is as evocative of summer as a tall, thirst-quenching glass of lemonade. This clean version adds a splash of sweet cherry juice for color and sweetness.

3½ cups plain tap or filtered water

2 cups ice

Juice from 2 lemons

½ cup 100 percent black cherry juice

4 TB. (¼ cup) agave nectar

Fresh mint leaves

Yield: 6 servings
Prep time: 10 minutes
Serving size: 1 cup
Each serving has:
59 calories
0 g total fat
0 g saturated fat
0 g protein
16 g carbohydrate
15 g sugars
0 mg cholesterol
0 g fiber
3 mg sodium

1. In a 2-quart pitcher add water, ice, lemon juice, cherry juice, and agave. Mix well, as agave tends to settle on the bottom.

2. Pour into tall glasses, garnish with mint, and serve.

Dirty Secrets

Sweet red cherries are usually of the Bing variety and are a dark purple-red color. Don't confuse them with sour cherries, which are the type used in pies. The most popular sour cherry is the Montmorency. Both sweet and sour cherry juices are available in natural food stores.

Breezy Blueberry Tea

Healthy green tea is the main component of this blueberry-flavored drink. Serve it hot or cold depending on your mood.

Yield: 3 servings
Prep time: 10 minutes
Serving size: 1 cup
Each serving has:
39 calories
0 g total fat
0 g saturated fat
0 g protein
10 g carbohydrate
7 g sugars
0 mg cholesterol
0 g fiber
6 mg sodium

2 cups plain tap or filtered water

2 green tea bags

¾ cup 100 percent natural wild blueberry juice

¼ cup orange juice

1. Heat water in a small saucepan over medium-high heat. When almost boiling (small bubbles begin to form), take off the heat and place tea bags in water. Steep for 4 minutes.

2. Remove tea bags from water. Pour into 1-quart pitcher. Add blueberry juice and orange juice. Pour over ice or serve hot.

Variation: You can make this tea with nearly any kind of fruit juice. Experiment with some of your favorites. Apple, peach, cherry, and raspberry are just a few options to consider.

Wholesome Habits

With no calories and half the caffeine in coffee, green tea is one of the healthiest beverages around. In China, where drinking tea originated, green tea is used as an elixir for everything from fighting infections to preventing heart disease.

Cranberry Apple Tea

This drink highlights the flavors of fall with tart cranberries, sweet apples, and rich black tea. Enjoy it any time of year.

4½ cups water

6 black tea bags

1 (3-inch) piece cinnamon stick

6 TB. 100 percent cranberry juice, unsweetened

1¼ cups apple cider

Yield: 8 servings
Prep time: 5 minutes
Serving size: 1 cup
Each serving has:
24 calories
0 g total fat
0 g saturated fat
0 g protein
6 g carbohydrate
5 g sugars
0 mg cholesterol
0 g fiber
3 mg sodium

1. Heat water in a small saucepan over medium-high heat. When almost boiling (small bubbles begin to form), take pot off the heat and place tea bags and cinnamon stick in water. Steep for 4 minutes.

2. Remove tea bags from water. Add cranberry juice and apple cider. Let sit for 5 minutes. Take out cinnamon stick. Serve warm or over ice.

Wholesome Habits

Aside from protecting you against urinary tract infections, scientists say vitamin C–rich cranberries can also reduce your risk of heart disease.

Part 4

Lovely Lunches

Whether you're brown-bagging it or eating in, the clean lunch recipes in the following chapters are sure to please.

You'll find imaginative salads—like Strawberry Spinach Salad, Greek Salmon Slaw, and Tropical Succotash—that are dressed with taste–bud–popping salad dressings made using natural juices, herbs, and spices to replace the fat and sugar.

The many savory sandwich recipes include cleaned up classics like our Italian Meatball Sub as well as innovations like Asian Turkey Sliders, which are wrapped in lettuce instead of bread.

And you can't talk about lunch without mentioning a bowl full of hearty soup! You'll learn how to prepare spectacular "cream" soups from puréed vegetables, as well as explore the world of beans, greens, and grains—all mainstays on the clean eating soup menu.

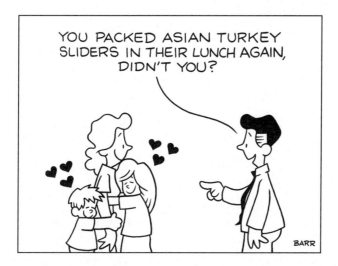

Chapter 13

Turning Over a New Leaf: Super Salads

In This Chapter

- ◆ Clean green recipes to live by
- ◆ Getting on the whole grain train
- ◆ Taking advantage of what the sea has to offer

When people think of eating clean and healthy, salads are often the first thing that comes to mind. And although it's true that chomping on a big bowl of leafy greens is good for you, for most people eating a salad is like walking through a minefield. Hidden dangers lie everywhere.

It's all too easy to load up on salty, fatty, highly processed ingredients like bacon bits, processed cheese, and preprepared tuna or chicken salad. Salad dressings are typically laden with mayonnaise and oils, often increasing the calorie count by hundreds. And finally, people tend to dole out giant portions for themselves.

We're here to show you that salads don't have to spell trouble. They can be clean, low-fat, healthy, and delicious, brimming with whole natural foods like vegetables, fruits, whole grains, and chicken or fish. You don't have to douse your salads in high-fat dressings to make them taste good, nor do you have to be a martyr and pucker up with just a sprinkle of lemon juice.

Our salad dressings pop with fresh herbs and spices and sing with simple fruit juices. Portions are just the right size to have you feeling satisfied without being bloated, and their fabulous colors and textures make them as beautiful to look at as they are to eat. So enjoy!

Chicken and Grapefruit Salad

Chicken and grapefruit may seem like an odd combination, but these two foods are perfectly suited for each other when combined with Middle Eastern spices and a cilantro almond dressing.

1 tsp. garlic powder

1 tsp. ground cinnamon

1 tsp. ground coriander

1 tsp. fresh ginger, grated

½ tsp. ground black pepper

12 oz. skinless, boneless chicken breast, thinly sliced

3 TB. nonfat plain yogurt

1 TB. onion, finely chopped

¼ cup all-natural, unsalted almond butter

1 TB. low-sodium tamari or 2 TB. low-sodium soy sauce

1 tsp. honey

½ tsp. hot sauce (optional)

2 large ruby red or pink grapefruits, peeled and sectioned (reserve juice)

2 TB. fresh cilantro, finely chopped

8 cups roughly chopped mixed greens (any combination of romaine, green leaf lettuce, and mixed baby greens)

Yield: 4 servings
Prep time: 20 minutes, plus 1 hour for marinating chicken
Cook time: 5 minutes
Serving size: 2 cups
Each serving has:
271 calories
11 g total fat
1 g saturated fat
25 g protein
21 g carbohydrate
6 g sugars
49 mg cholesterol
4 g fiber
341 mg sodium

1. In a small bowl mix garlic powder, cinnamon, coriander, ginger, and black pepper until well blended. Sprinkle on chicken and toss to coat. Add yogurt and onion. Mix well. Marinate chicken for at least 1 hour in the refrigerator or overnight. Chicken can be prepared a day in advance.

2. After chicken has marinated, heat oven to broil on high. In a medium bowl whisk together almond butter, tamari, honey, and hot sauce (if using) until smooth and creamy. Add ⅓ cup of reserved grapefruit juice or enough to make a smooth thin dressing. Sprinkle in cilantro. Mix well.

3. Line a cookie sheet with foil and lightly coat foil with cooking spray. Place marinated spiced chicken on cookie sheet and broil in oven for 5 minutes.

4. To assemble, on each plate place 2 cups lettuce, grapefruit sections (about ⅓ cup for each serving), 3 ounces spiced chicken, and drizzle with 2 to 3 tablespoons dressing. Makes 4 plates. Serve immediately.

Clean Cuts

To section a grapefruit, place fruit on flat, clean work surface. Cut off both ends and place flat side down. Next cut off outside skin and white pith, leaving only fruit. Then cut fruit on both sides along each section to the center (like a triangle) and pop fruit section out. (To save the juice, after removing the pith section the fruit over a small bowl.)

Whole Wheat Italian Bread Salad

Italians call this *Panzanella* salad, and they created it to use up left-over bread, but it's so good you'll want to buy an extra loaf just to make it. It's best made in the summer when basil and tomatoes are at their peak.

5 oz. day old whole wheat bread, cut into ½-inch cubes (about 5 slices of bread about ½-inch thick)

1 lb. medium tomatoes (3–4 medium tomatoes), cored, seeded, and diced

1 large roasted red bell pepper, finely chopped

1 cup cooked white beans

1 garlic clove, peeled and minced

2 TB. kalamata olives, finely chopped

2 TB. extra-virgin olive oil

2 TB. fresh basil, finely chopped

1 TB. white balsamic vinegar or white wine vinegar

Juice from ½ lemon

¼ tsp. ground black pepper

1 oz. feta cheese

Yield: 4 servings
Prep time: 15 minutes
Serving size: 1 cup
Each serving has:
265 calories
12 g total fat
3 g saturated fat
11 g protein
31 g carbohydrate
7 g sugars
6 mg cholesterol
7 g fiber
300 mg sodium

1. In a large bowl toss whole wheat bread, tomatoes, red pepper, white beans, garlic, and kalamata olives. Let sit for 15 minutes so flavors can blend.

2. In a small bowl, whisk together olive oil, basil, vinegar, lemon juice, and black pepper. Pour over bread salad and gently mix together. Sprinkle with feta cheese. Serve.

Variation: Aside from bread and tomatoes, this salad can be made with just about anything. Try varying the beans (chickpeas work well), or excluding them altogether. As for vegetables, try carrots, celery, cucumber, red onion, or whatever you have on hand. You might even want to use flavored bread such as sun-dried tomato or garlic whole wheat bread.

Clean Meanings

Panzanella is the Italian name for this tomato-bread salad that originated around Tuscany. Although bread is the basic ingredient, the real focus is on fresh, seasonal summer vegetables.

Strawberry Spinach Salad with Feta

Sweet strawberries and tender baby spinach tossed with a lemony poppy seed dressing make this salad a winner any time. Serve it when you want to impress guests or when you just want a special treat.

Yield: 4 servings
Prep time: 15 minutes
Serving size: 2 cups
Each serving has:
144 calories
11 g total fat
3 g saturated fat
5 g protein
8 g carbohydrate
4 g sugars
12 mg cholesterol
2 g fiber
399 mg sodium

4 oz. (about 6 cups) baby spinach, washed and dried

1 cup fresh sliced strawberries

1 cup sliced and halved cucumber

2 tsp. lemon zest

2 tsp. lemon juice

2 TB. extra-virgin olive oil

¼ tsp. sea salt

¼ tsp. ground black pepper

2 tsp. Dijon mustard

2 garlic cloves, peeled and crushed

4 TB. low-fat plain Greek yogurt

4 tsp. apple cider vinegar

2 TB. low-sodium chicken stock

2 TB. fresh basil, finely chopped

1 tsp. poppy seeds

2 oz. feta, crumbled

1. Place 1½ cups spinach on each of four large dinner plates. Top each with ¼ cup strawberries and ¼ cup cucumber. Set aside.

2. In a small bowl whisk lemon zest, lemon juice, olive oil, salt, black pepper, mustard, garlic, yogurt, vinegar, chicken stock, and basil until light and frothy. Stir in poppy seeds and beat until blended. Divide and pour over top of spinach-strawberry-cucumber salad (about 3 tablespoons for each). Sprinkle with crumbled feta and serve.

Wholesome Habits _____

Popeye was right. Spinach is a super food. For only a few calories, it offers an impressive array of vitamins and minerals and particularly high levels of vitamin K, vitamin A, the B vitamin folate, the minerals magnesium and manganese, and several carotenoids.

Greek Salmon Slaw

Imagine yourself soaking up the sun on a Greek island when you eat this salad spiked with lemon, oregano, and garlic. Broccoli, carrots, and red cabbage keep it light, while the salmon boasts heart-healthy omega-3 fatty acids.

4 (3-oz.) salmon filets, skinned

1 (12-oz.) bag of broccoli slaw

4 TB. red pepper or tomato, diced

4 tsp. red onion, diced

2 tsp. fresh oregano, finely chopped

1 garlic clove, peeled and crushed

1 tsp. lemon zest

2 tsp. lemon juice

4 tsp. extra-virgin olive oil

1 tsp. white balsamic vinegar or white wine vinegar

¼ tsp. ground black pepper

⅛ tsp. sea salt

Pinch cayenne pepper, optional

Yield: 4 servings
Prep time: 10 minutes
Cook time: 7 minutes
Serving size: 1 cup slaw plus 3 ounces of salmon
Each serving has:
198 calories
16 g total fat
3 g saturated fat
20 g protein
7 g carbohydrate
3 g sugars
47 mg cholesterol
3 g fiber
149 mg sodium

1. Heat oven to high broil. Place broccoli slaw, red pepper, and red onion in a large bowl. Toss together.

2. In a medium bowl whisk together oregano, garlic, lemon zest, lemon juice, olive oil, white balsamic vinegar, black pepper, sea salt, and cayenne (if using).

3. Pour dressing over broccoli slaw mixture and toss to coat. Let sit for 5 to 10 minutes.

4. Place salmon on stoneware or cookie sheet covered with foil and sprayed with cooking spray. Broil on high for 5 to 6 minutes.

5. To assemble, place 1 cup slaw on each dinner plate, top with 3 ounces of salmon, and serve.

Clean Cuts

If you can't find broccoli slaw in the produce section, just make your own. In a food processor, shred 8 ounces of peeled broccoli stems (save the crowns for another time), 2 ounces of carrot, and 2 ounces of red cabbage. Toss together and store in an airtight container in the refrigerator.

Tropical Shrimp Succotash

Traditional succotash is a mixture of corn and lima beans. Here we keep the corn but add *edamame* beans, mango, and shrimp, all dressed with Asian-inspired ingredients.

Yield: 4 servings
Prep time: 10 minutes
Cook time: 5 minutes
Serving size: 1 cup
Each serving has:
210 calories
8 g total fat
1 g saturated fat
19 g protein
17 g carbohydrate
10 g sugars
109 mg cholesterol
4 g fiber
204 mg sodium

2 cups edamame, cooked from frozen and shelled (can substitute cooked baby lima beans)

8 oz. large cooked shrimp (31–40 count), tail off, cut into bite-sized pieces (about 18 shrimp)

1 large mango, diced, or 1 cup mandarin oranges in natural fruit juice, drained

¼ cup frozen corn, thawed

4 tsp. green onion, chopped

2 tsp. sesame seed oil

½ tsp. chili paste or hot sauce

2 tsp. rice vinegar

1 tsp. lime juice

2 tsp. canola oil

2 tsp. fresh *galangal* or ginger root, peeled and finely chopped

1 tsp. low-sodium *tamari* sauce

1 tsp. unsweetened shredded coconut

1. Follow package directions to cook edamame, omitting salt.

2. In large bowl, toss together shrimp, mango, edamame, corn, and green onion.

3. In a small bowl whisk sesame seed oil, chili paste, rice vinegar, lime juice, canola oil, galangal, and tamari until blended.

4. Pour dressing over shrimp. Toss together. Let sit for 5 to 10 minutes. Sprinkle with coconut. Can be served cold or at room temperature.

Clean Meanings

Galangal is known as Thai ginger. It looks similar to ginger but has a milder taste. Galangal is available at Asian grocery stores, but ginger will work just as well in recipes. **Edamame** are fresh green soybeans; they taste sweet and clean. Although you can find them shelled they're most often sold frozen in their inedible pod. **Tamari** is a darker thicker version of soy sauce with a more intense flavor.

Fruity Couscous Salad

Raisins, apples, and green peas give whole wheat couscous color as well as flavor in this surprisingly simple cold salad.

2 cups water	**1 TB. olive oil**
1 cup whole wheat couscous	**1 large garlic clove, peeled and crushed**
3 TB. seedless raisins	**2 TB. orange juice**
¾ cup frozen peas, thawed	**1½ tsp. orange zest**
¾ cup apple (about 1 small), cored and diced	**2 TB. fresh parsley, finely chopped**
3 TB. red onion, diced	**1 TB. fresh mint, finely chopped**
¾ tsp. curry powder	

Yield: 3 servings
Prep time: 10 minutes
Serving size: 1½ cups
Each serving has:
324 calories
6 g total fat
1 g saturated fat
9 g protein
61 g carbohydrate
12 g sugars
0 mg cholesterol
9 g fiber
42 mg sodium

1. In a small saucepan heat water until boiling. Add couscous, raisins, peas, apple, red onion, and curry powder. Remove from heat. Stir once. Cover and let sit for about 6 minutes or until couscous is cooked through.

2. In a small bowl, whisk together olive oil, garlic, orange juice, orange zest, parsley, and mint.

3. When couscous is done, transfer to a bowl and let cool for 5 to 10 minutes. Pour on dressing and gently toss to mix. Salad can be eaten warm or cold.

Variation: Almost any combination of dried fruit (dried cherries, cranberries, or dates, for instance) and fresh fruit (try oranges, strawberries, or peaches) will work in this salad. To make it a main dish, mix in 1 cup cooked beans such as chickpeas, kidney beans, or white beans or 1 cup cooked chicken or pork.

Wholesome Habits

Couscous (a small wheat pasta) is a mainstay in Moroccan cuisine where it traditionally serves as the base for a variety of meat or vegetable stews. Most couscous is refined and yellow in color, but whole wheat (brown) couscous is now available.

White Beans and Mixed Greens

Creamy white beans and basil complement the dark leafy greens beautifully.

Yield: 4 servings
Prep time: 10 minutes
Serving size: 3 cups mixed greens plus ½ cup beans
Each serving has:
148 calories
7 g total fat
1 g saturated fat
6 g protein
16 g carbohydrate
2 g sugars
0 mg cholesterol
6 g fiber
66 mg sodium

1 cup cooked white beans

2 TB. celery, chopped

1 TB. red onion, chopped

¼ cup tomato, small diced

½ cup packed fresh basil

2 TB. extra-virgin olive oil

1 TB. plus 1 tsp. white balsamic vinegar or white wine vinegar

2 TB. low-sodium chicken stock

1 small garlic clove, peeled and coarsely chopped

⅛ tsp. ground black pepper

⅛ tsp. sea salt

12 cups mixed field greens

1. In a small bowl, mix white beans, celery, red onion, and tomato. Set aside.

2. Place basil, olive oil, vinegar, chicken stock, and garlic in mini food processor. Process on high for about 30 seconds. Stop and scrape down sides with rubber spatula. Process for 10 more seconds or until smooth.

3. Pour dressing over beans. Sprinkle with pepper and salt. Let marinate for 10 to 15 minutes.

4. Right before serving, toss white beans with mixed greens. Serve 3-cup portions on dinner plates.

Clean Cuts _____

Since lettuce has such high water content, it contains few calories and is a great addition on clean menus. To boost nutritional value, go for dark leaf varieties.

Savory Sandwiches

In This Chapter

- ◆ Cleaning up old stand-bys
- ◆ Boosting flavor without salt, sugar, or fat
- ◆ It's all about the bread

Even though the invention of the sandwich is credited to an Englishman who was too busy to stop playing cards to eat, these hand-held meals are about as American as apple pie—and as popular. For lunch, one out of every three meals is a sandwich. We love them so much we've even given them special names like submarines, grinders, hoagies, heroes, and po' boys. Unfortunately, these gargantuan sandwiches are typically loaded with fat and salt, thanks to fatty meats, lots of cheese, and rich spreads.

In this chapter we've trimmed down the calories by cutting down—and sometimes even cutting out—the cheese, choosing lean meats, and watching portion size. Don't worry: we haven't skimped on fillings. You'll be amazed at how hearty these sandwiches are.

We've gone crazy boosting sandwiches with dried fruits, vegetables, and whole grains to create an explosion of clean flavors while still controlling calories.

And just because it's a sandwich doesn't mean it has to use two slices of whole wheat bread. We'll introduce you to wraps, pitas, and Ezekiel bread. There's even a recipe for Asian-inspired turkey burgers wrapped in lettuce leaves. Varying the type of bread (or not having bread at all) offers you an endless array of possibilities. It also helps keep sodium levels down. Considering that bread is the source of much of the sodium in the American diet, it pays to be creative. Man cannot live by bread or sandwiches alone, but they sure do hit the spot sometimes.

Regal Roast Beef Sandwiches

Instead of slathering this classic roast beef sandwich with mayonnaise, it's dressed with a yogurt-horseradish-garlic-rosemary spread. With so much flavor, you won't miss the fat.

1 garlic clove, peeled and crushed

¼ cup nonfat, plain Greek yogurt

2 TB. low-fat sour cream

1 heaping tsp. fresh rosemary leaves, finely chopped

1 tsp. prepared horseradish

⅛ tsp. kosher salt

⅛ tsp. ground black pepper

8 slices Italian whole wheat bread

12 oz. cooked roast beef, bottom round or eye round, thinly sliced (see recipe in Chapter 17)

8 thin tomato slices

8 small lettuce leaves

Yield: 4 sandwiches
Prep time: 10 minutes
Serving size: 1 sandwich
Each serving has:
295 calories
5 g total fat
2 g saturated fat
27 g protein
38 g carbohydrate
4 g sugars
45 mg cholesterol
4 g fiber
481 mg sodium

1. In a small bowl, add crushed garlic, yogurt, sour cream, rosemary, horseradish, salt, and pepper. Mix well. Set aside.

2. Place 4 slices of bread on a work surface and spread each with 1 tablespoon of yogurt sauce. Top with 3 ounces of roast beef, 2 slices of tomato, and 2 lettuce leaves, and place remaining 4 slices of bread on top of each. Slice each sandwich in half and serve.

Variation: For a hot version of this sandwich, replace the lettuce and tomato with 2 tablespoons sautéd peppers and onions for each sandwich. Heat the meat and bread in the oven, then add the sauce.

Dirty Secrets

This recipe uses cooked fresh meat. Try to avoid deli meats. Not only are they high in sodium, sugar, and fat and contain all sorts of preservatives and additives, they're also expensive. You can create your own clean deli-style meats by cooking fresh meats and investing in a good slicer.

Asian Turkey Sliders

These mini burgers include traditional Asian flavors—green onion, ginger, garlic, homemade hoisin sauce, and wasabi. To keep calories and sodium under control, we've ditched the bread and wrapped them in lettuce leaves.

Yield: 4 servings
(8 mini burgers)

Prep time: 10 minutes
Cook time: 25 minutes
Serving size: 2 mini burgers

Each serving has:
171 calories
8 g total fat
2 g saturated fat
16 g protein
9 g carbohydrate
1 g sugars
66 mg cholesterol
1 g fiber
166 mg sodium

12 oz. (93 percent lean) ground turkey

1 tsp. garlic clove, peeled and crushed

2 TB. green onion, chopped

½ tsp. grated fresh ginger

½ cup cooked short grain brown rice

4 tsp. Homemade Hoisin Sauce (see recipe in Chapter 22)

¼ tsp. Chinese five-spice powder

1 tsp. wasabi paste

8 butterhead or romaine lettuce leaves

1. Heat oven to 375°F. In a large bowl mix ground turkey, garlic, green onion, ginger, rice, hoisin sauce, five-spice powder, and wasabi paste with a wooden spoon or your hands.

2. Shape meat into 8 (2-ounce) patties. Place on a baking stone or a cookie sheet covered with aluminum foil and sprayed with cooking spray.

3. Bake for 25 minutes or until juices run clear when meat is poked with a fork. The meat should register 165°F when probed with a meat thermometer.

4. To serve, put lettuce leaf on flat work surface and place ground turkey patty at the bottom of the leaf. Roll up, tucking ends in as you go. Serve with Mango Pineapple Salsa (recipe in Chapter 11).

Dirty Secrets

Check the label on ground turkey. You want to choose turkey that's labeled at least 93 percent lean or extra-lean and contains ground turkey breast. If it just says "ground turkey" you're getting fatty dark meat and skin along with breast meat.

Loaded Black Bean Burrito

You can't go wrong with this tasty black bean burrito. It's bursting with fiber and colorful, good-for-you ingredients.

1 (8-inch) whole wheat tortilla

¼ cup cooked black or red beans drained and rinsed (cooked with no salt)

¼ cup cooked brown rice

2 TB. corn, fresh cooked or thawed from frozen

1 TB. low-sodium salsa

1 TB. low-fat sour cream

1 TB. Clean Tomato Avocado Corn Salsa (see recipe in Chapter 12)

2 tsp. reduced-fat Mexican cheese blend

Hot sauce (optional)

Yield: 1 serving
Prep time: 5 minutes
Serving size: 1 burrito
Each serving has:
322 calories
8 g total fat
2 g saturated fat
12 g protein
53 g carbohydrate
4 g sugars
11 mg cholesterol
9 g fiber
509 mg sodium

1. For easier rolling, warm tortilla in a large skillet over medium heat for about 30 seconds per side, or warm, wrapped in damp paper towel, in a microwave oven for 15 to 20 seconds.

2. To assemble, place tortilla on a large flat cutting board or work surface. Spread black beans down center and top half of tortilla, leaving a 1½-inch border. Top beans with cooked brown rice, corn, salsa, sour cream, and tomato-avocado salsa (in that order). Sprinkle with cheese and a few drops of hot sauce (if using).

3. Fold the two sides in about 2 inches, then roll the tortilla to enclose the bean mixture. Serve immediately or wrap tightly in plastic wrap and store in refrigerator; wrap will keep for 2 to 3 days. To serve from refrigerator, reheat in microwave for 20 or 30 seconds.

Clean Cuts

If you don't have the Clean Tomato Avocado Corn Salsa prepared, make a quick version from scratch. Simply mix 1 tablespoon chopped tomato, 1 tablespoon chopped avocado, and 1 teaspoon chopped cilantro with a squeeze of lime juice and a pinch of salt.

The Ultimate Tuna Salad Sandwich

Dried cranberries and a hard-boiled egg bring this tuna salad sandwich to new heights. They also help stretch your dollars.

Yield: 2 servings
Prep time: 10 minutes
Serving size: 1 sandwich (½ cup tuna salad)
Each serving has:
372 calories
9 g total fat
3 g saturated fat
32 g protein
41 g carbohydrate
5 g sugars
314 mg cholesterol
5 g fiber
467 mg sodium

4 oz. fresh yellowfin tuna

1 large hard-boiled egg, shelled

1 TB. celery, finely chopped

1 TB. green onion, finely chopped

1 TB. dried cranberries, chopped

¼ cup plus 1 TB. plain nonfat yogurt

½ tsp. fresh thyme leaves, finely chopped

2 large whole wheat pitas (6½ inches in diameter)

8 leaves fresh watercress

1. Heat a small sauté pan over medium heat until hot. Spray with cooking spray and place tuna in pan. Cook 2 to 3 minutes on each side depending on thickness, until all pink has disappeared from fish. Set aside on plate.

2. In a small bowl, mash hard-boiled egg with a fork; add celery, green onion, cranberries, yogurt, and thyme.

3. Break tuna up on plate with fork until shredded. Add tuna to egg-yogurt mixture and mix until well blended.

4. Cut each pita in half, open the pocket up and place two watercress leaves inside each half of pita. Add ¼ cup tuna-cranberry salad to each half pita pocket. One serving is two half pita pockets.

Wholesome Habits

The five most popular varieties of tuna are yellowfin, bluefin, bigeye, skipjack, and albacore. Yellowfin is also known by its Hawaiian name, ahi, and is most commonly available fresh; bluefin is the most prized and most expensive tuna in the world (usually served raw); bigeye is also served raw in sushi or sashimi; skipjack is what's found in a can except when labeled premium white meat, which is albacore.

Italian Meatball Sub

Zesty Italian seasonings liven up these lean meatballs while roasted red pepper and bulgur are the secret ingredients that keep them moist. Dressed with sauce and cheese you'll never know they're low calorie.

½ large red pepper, seeded

1 lb. (93 percent lean) ground beef

2 TB. fresh basil, finely chopped

1 tsp. fresh oregano, finely chopped

2 slices whole wheat bread, crust removed, sprinkled with 3 TB. water

2 garlic cloves, peeled and minced

¼ tsp. ground black pepper

¼ cup fine bulgur soaked in 1 cup warm water for 10 minutes

4 TB. grated Parmesan cheese

9 whole wheat rolls

1¼ cup no salt added tomato sauce or Basic Tomato Sauce (see recipe in Chapter 17)

9 TB. shredded low-fat mozzarella

Yield: 9 servings
Prep time: 20 minutes
Cook time: 25 minutes
Serving size: 1 sandwich (3 meatballs each plus sauce and cheese and roll)
Each serving has:
333 calories
9 g total fat
4 g saturated fat
22 g protein
43 g carbohydrate
8 g sugars
42 mg cholesterol
7 g fiber
498 mg sodium

1. Heat oven to 450°F, place ½ pepper, skin side up, on a baking stone or cookie sheet covered with aluminum foil and lightly coated with cooking spray. Bake for 20 minutes. Remove from oven, lower the oven temperature to 375°F, and set pepper on plate to cool.

2. Meanwhile in a large bowl, combine ground beef, basil, oregano, soaked whole wheat bread, garlic, and black pepper with a wooden spoon or by hand.

3. Drain water from bulgur. When red pepper is cool, remove stem, seeds, and skin, and finely chop. Mix red pepper, bulgur, and Parmesan cheese into ground beef and blend thoroughly.

4. Cover a baking sheet with aluminum foil sprayed with cooking spray. Form ground beef into 1-ounce balls using a 1-ounce scoop (about the size of a golf ball). Place on cookie sheet or stone. You should have about 27 meatballs.

5. Bake at 375°F for 25 minutes.

6. On a flat work surface, slice Italian whole wheat rolls in half. To assemble, place 3 meatballs in each roll, cover with 2 table-spoons of tomato sauce and sprinkle with 1 tablespoon of mozzarella cheese. For a hot sandwich, place under broiler for 1 minute until cheese melts.

Clean Cuts

Cook up a big batch of these meatballs. Let them cool, then portion them up and freeze them in large freezer bags. Take them out any time you need to prepare a quick meal. They make a great addition to soups or paired with whole wheat pasta.

Grilled Chicken Sandwich

This sandwich is simple and delicious. Dressed with creamy avocado and a sweet spicy orange sauce, it can easily be served for
dinner as well as lunch. Plus, the high-fiber bread fills you up.
For a complete meal, serve with Apples and Nuts (see recipe in
Chapter 9) and a Trail Mix Cookie (see recipe in Chapter 23).

**3½ oz. chicken breast,
pounded thin**

2 slices *Ezekiel 4:9 bread*

**1½ TB. Orange Agave Sauce
(see recipe in Chapter 22)**

2 slices avocado (about 1 oz.)

1 slice tomato

¼ cup shredded lettuce

Yield: 1 serving
Prep time: 10 minutes
Serving size: 1 sandwich
Each serving has:
358 calories
7 g total fat
2 g saturated fat
31 g protein
42 g carbohydrate
8 g sugars
57 mg cholesterol
8 g fiber
247 mg sodium

1. Heat small sauté pan over medium-high heat. Spray with
   cooking spray. Place chicken breast in pan and cook about
   3 minutes on each side, or until juices run clear when poked
   with a fork.

2. To assemble, place one slice of bread on a flat work surface.
   Top with chicken breast. Spread orange agave sauce over
   chicken, then add avocado, tomato, and shredded lettuce. Top
   with remaining slice of bread. Cut sandwich in half and serve.

Variation: For a simple twist, replace the orange agave sauce with
1 tablespoon all-natural fruit-sweetened apricot or peach preserves
mixed with ¼ teaspoon finely chopped jalapeño and a dash of
ground cloves.

Clean Meanings

Ezekiel 4:9 bread is a 100 percent whole grain bread
made from 6 sprouted organic grains and legumes—whole
wheat, malted barley, whole millet, whole barley, whole lentils,
whole soybeans, and whole spelt. Sprouting the grains makes
the bread more easily digestible and improves the protein quality. It's low in sodium and has a low glycemic index, meaning it
won't cause blood sugar levels to spike. Ezekiel bread can be
found in the frozen section of natural or whole food stores.

Chapter 15

Sensational Soups

In This Chapter

- ◆ Creamy creations without cream and butter
- ◆ The best of the bean soups
- ◆ Revisiting the classics
- ◆ Clean soups you can count on

There's nothing more comforting or satisfying than a big bowl of home-made soup. It's hearty, delicious, and, when prepared with the right ingredients, as nutritious as it gets. No wonder soup is a staple on clean eating menus.

The recipes in this chapter use fresh vegetables, whole grains, and beans. Since these soups don't rely on heavy cream or butter for flavor—vegetable purées or homemade broths make-up their base—fat and calories are kept to a minimum.

Sodium levels are kept in check with homemade vegetable, chicken, or beef stocks (more about preparing these in Chapter 17), but if you're short on time or don't have any around, low-sodium canned broths are always an option (keep in mind that even low-sodium brands are still higher in sodium than homemade).

A Weighty Advantage

There's one more reason you'll want to include homemade soups in your clean eating repertoire: weight loss. Studies show that people who eat a cup of broth or vegetable-based soup prior to their meal (say, as a first course) eat less food overall for the day than those who don't dine on soup. Fewer calories mean fewer pounds on you, making it easier to maintain a healthy figure.

Dirty Secrets

Avoid any store-bought processed or preprepared soups, even if they look clean. Read the label and you're likely to find hidden sugar and salt.

So, what's soup have over other low-calorie foods? It's filling and satisfying. Keeping calories in check is simple, too. All the soups in this chapter, including rich and creamy Crab and Butternut Squash Bisque and Hearty Onion Soup, have fewer than 200 calories a serving.

Soup Is Good Food

On the culinary side, soups can make your life a lot less complicated. First of all you don't have to be a whiz in the kitchen to make them. Most take only a few simple ingredients and a good stock to make their magic, and many can be whipped up within a half hour. They also work great with leftovers.

Even if you have a small family or are single, make the entire soup recipe (they were written to make several servings). This way you can keep a batch on hand in the refrigerator or freezer to pull out for a quick weekday dinner, a filling snack, or as an appetizer or side dish with part of your meal. Stocking up on soup means you'll always have a healthy, substantial, and satisfying meal available at any time.

Crab and Butternut Squash *Bisque*

This sweet butternut squash soup, thickened with cooked brown rice, is complemented by a colorful garnish of crabmeat, tomato, and avocado.

4 cups Baked Butternut Squash (see recipe in Chapter 19)

2 tsp. fresh thyme leaves, finely chopped

3½ cups Homemade Chicken Stock (see recipe in Chapter 17) or low-sodium canned

½ cup cooked brown rice

1 cup low-fat milk

¼ tsp. ground black pepper

8 oz. cooked blue crabmeat

½ medium (about 3½ oz.) avocado, peeled, pitted, and finely diced

7 TB. tomato, finely chopped (about ½ medium tomato)

Yield: 7 servings
Prep time: 10 minutes
Cook time: 10 minutes
Serving size: 1 cup
Each serving has:
174 calories
4 g total fat
1 g saturated fat
12 g protein
25 g carbohydrate
6 g sugars
34 mg cholesterol
4 g fiber
149 mg sodium

1. Place butternut squash, thyme, chicken stock, brown rice, milk, and black pepper in a large saucepan over medium-high heat. Bring to a boil. Reduce heat to a simmer (low heat), cover, and cook for 8 minutes.

2. Pour mixture into a blender and purée for 30 seconds or until smooth.

3. Pour 1 cup of soup into each serving bowl. Top each bowl with about 1 tablespoon crabmeat, 1 tablespoon tomato, and about 1 tablespoon avocado. Serve immediately.

Clean Meanings

Bisque is a French word that describes a rich, creamy soup, usually made with heavy cream and seafood. In this recipe we've eliminated the cream, added puréed squash, and included seafood in the garnish.

Pumpkin and Wild Mushroom Soup

Earthy wild mushrooms give this smooth, glossy pumpkin soup flavor and texture. Low-fat milk makes for a creamy finish. Complement this soup with a green salad and a whole wheat roll for a complete meal.

Yield: 8 servings
Prep time: 10 minutes
Cook time: 20 minutes
Serving size: 1 cup
Each serving has:
76 calories
2 g total fat
0 g saturated fat
5 g protein
10 g carbohydrate
5 g sugars
2 mg cholesterol
2 g fiber
211 mg sodium

2 tsp. olive oil

1 garlic clove, peeled and minced

½ small onion, diced into ¼-inch pieces

½ cup celery, diced (1 medium stalk)

2 green onions, diced

3 cups sliced wild mushrooms (mixture of cremini, shiitakes, portobello, and oysters)

1 (15-oz.) can pumpkin

4 cups Homemade Chicken Stock (see recipe in Chapter 17) or low-sodium canned

1 cup water

2 tsp. fresh thyme leaves, finely chopped

½ tsp. sea salt

¼ tsp. ground black pepper

2 tsp. sherry or red wine

1 cup low-fat (1 percent) milk

1. Heat olive oil over medium-high heat in a 4-quart stock pot. Add garlic, onion, celery, green onion, and mushrooms. Cook for 4 to 5 minutes or until soft.

2. Add pumpkin, chicken stock, and water. Cover and bring to a boil. Add thyme, salt, pepper, and sherry. Lower the heat to a simmer and cook for 10 minutes.

3. Remove from heat and slowly whisk in milk. Serve immediately.

Variation: For a heartier soup, add 2 cups Wild Rice Blend (see recipe in Chapter 20) and 1 cup cooked, diced pork.

Clean Cuts

This recipe uses exotic or wild mushrooms like cremini, Italian browns, portobellos, shiitakes, and oyster mushrooms, but you can also make it with all white domestic mushrooms (or any combination of mushrooms).

Golden Carrot Soup

Yukon Gold potatoes make this soup smooth and buttery while pineapple juice and ginger bring out the sweetness of the carrots.

2 tsp. olive oil

2 cups fresh carrots, peeled and cut into 1-inch pieces (4 medium carrots)

½ small onion, chopped

2 garlic cloves, peeled and minced

1 medium Yukon Gold potato, diced (about 1 cup)

3 cups Homemade Chicken Stock (see recipe in Chapter 17) or low-sodium canned

1 cup pineapple juice

¼ tsp. sea salt (optional)

¼ tsp. ground black pepper

½ tsp. fresh ginger, peeled and grated

Pinch of nutmeg

½ cup low-fat (1 percent) milk

Yield: 4 servings
Prep time: 20 minutes
Cook time: 30 minutes
Serving size: 1 cup
Each serving has:
158 calories
4 g total fat
1 g saturated fat
6 g protein
27 g carbohydrate
12 g sugars
2 mg cholesterol
3 g fiber
116 mg sodium

1. Heat olive oil in a 4-quart pot over medium-high heat. Add carrot, onion, and garlic and sauté about 5 minutes or until onion begins to turn translucent.

2. Add potato, chicken stock, and pineapple juice. Bring to a boil, lower the heat to medium-low, and simmer covered for 20 to 25 minutes until carrots are tender.

3. Pour soup mixture in blender and purée for 1 minute. Pour back in pot, and place over medium heat. Add salt (if using), black pepper, ginger, and nutmeg. Stir. After about a minute slowly add low-fat milk. Heat through (about 3 minutes). Serve immediately.

Variation: For a vegan version of this recipe, substitute vegetable broth for the chicken stock and replace the low-fat milk with unsweetened soymilk.

Wholesome Habits

Carrots keep your eyes in tip top shape, thanks to high levels of beta-carotene, a precursor to vitamin A. Beta-carotene is essential for night vision and protects eyes from macular degeneration (an eye disease that can cause blindness late in life) and cataracts.

Swiss Chard and Kidney Bean Soup

This is the kind of hearty soup—filled with beans, Swiss chard, and quinoa—that you'd make on a rainy day. Our Eating Clean Spice Blend gives it a savory, spicy kick and quinoa supplies texture, fiber, and nuttiness.

Yield: 8 cups
Prep time: 10 minutes
Cook time: 15 to 20 minutes
Serving size: 1 cup
Each serving has:
101 calories
2 g total fat
0 g saturated fat
4 g protein
18 g carbohydrate
2 g sugars
0 mg cholesterol
3 g fiber
125 mg sodium

Wholesome Habits

In the food world beans are nutritional superstars. They're rich in protein, folate, and several minerals. They also consistently rank higher in antioxidants than most fruits and vegetables. Healthwise they've been linked to lower risks of heart disease, cancer, and diabetes.

1 tsp. olive oil

½ medium onion, small diced

1 garlic clove, peeled and minced

½ cup quinoa

1 cup cooked red kidney beans, drained and rinsed

4 cups fresh Swiss chard (or other leafy green spinachlike vegetable), roughly chopped

2 tsp. Eating Clean Spice Blend (see recipe in Chapter 21)

2 tsp. Eating Clean Herb Paste (see recipe in Chapter 21) or 1 TB. fresh oregano leaves, chopped

¼ tsp. sea salt

⅛ tsp. cracked black pepper

6 cups Roasted Vegetable Stock or Homemade Chicken Stock (see recipe in Chapter 17) or low-sodium canned

Parmesan cheese (optional)

1. Heat olive oil in a 4-quart pot over medium-high heat. Sauté onion and garlic for about 2 minutes. Add quinoa, stirring for about a minute until toasty brown.

2. Add kidney beans, Swiss chard, spice blend, herb paste, salt, pepper, and vegetable broth. Bring to a boil. Cover and reduce heat to a simmer. Cook for about 10 minutes. Quinoa will turn translucent.

3. Serve immediately. If using Parmesan cheese, sprinkle ½ teaspoon on top of each soup bowl before serving.

Variation: Don't hesitate to change up the beans and/or the greens in this recipe. Try white beans and escarole or pinto beans and spinach instead of the Swiss chard and kidney beans. Mix and match any combination of beans and greens.

Lentil and Kale Soup

Kale gives a splash of color to this hearty and nutrient-packed soup, while lemon zest and tamari add some zing.

1 TB. olive oil

3 garlic cloves, peeled and minced

1 cup onion, chopped

½ cup celery, chopped (1 medium stalk)

¾ cup carrot, diced (1 medium)

1 (1-lb.) bag of dried brown lentils, rinsed and picked over for stones

6 cups Homemade Chicken Stock (see recipe in Chapter 17) or low-sodium canned

4 cups water

1 (10-oz.) bunch kale, chopped (can substitute mustard greens, Swiss chard, spinach, or any other cooking green)

1 large tomato, chopped

¼ tsp. ground black pepper

¾ tsp. kosher salt

1 TB. low-sodium tamari

1 tsp. lemon zest

2 TB. fresh parsley, finely chopped

2 TB. fresh basil, finely chopped

Yield: 12 servings
Prep time: 30 minutes
Cook time: 1 hour
Serving size: 1 cup
Each serving has:
188 calories
3 g total fat
0 g saturated fat
14 g protein
30 g carbohydrate
2 g sugars
0 mg cholesterol
13 g fiber
236 mg sodium

1. Heat olive oil in a 4-quart stockpot over medium-high heat. Add garlic, onion, celery, and carrot. Cook for 4 to 5 minutes or until soft.

2. Add lentils, chicken stock, and water. Cover and bring to a boil. Lower the heat to a simmer and cook for 30 minutes.

3. Add kale, tomato, pepper, salt, tamari, lemon zest, basil, and parsley. Simmer for another 30 minutes.

4. For a smoother soup, take out two cups of soup and purée in blender or food processor, then mix back in.

5. Serve hot with whole wheat rolls or over brown rice.

Wholesome Habits

Unlike dried beans, lentils (classified as legumes) need no presoaking. They come in a range of colors from yellow and orange to deep red, green, and black. In India, where they are a staple, people eat lentils twice a day.

Marvelous *Minestrone*

Basic pantry and refrigerator staples—celery, onions, carrots, beans, and tomato—combine with classic Italian seasonings for this soup. It's perfect when time is short. Make a big batch to freeze for later on.

Yield: 10 servings
Prep time: 10 minutes
Cook time: 25 minutes
Serving size: 1 cup
Each serving has:
119 calories
3 g total fat
1 g saturated fat
6 g protein
18 g carbohydrate
4 g sugars
1 mg cholesterol
4 g fiber
118 mg sodium

Clean Meanings

Minestrone comes from the Italian word *minestra,* which means soup. Minestrone, or "big soup," refers to its hearty character— a combination of beans, rice or pasta, and vegetables.

1 medium onion, diced (about ½ cup)

1 medium stalk celery, diced (about ½ cup)

1 small carrot, diced (about ½ cup)

2 small zucchinis, diced (about 2 cups)

2 garlic cloves, peeled and minced

2 tsp. olive oil

5 cups Homemade Chicken Stock (see recipe in Chapter 17) or low-sodium canned

3 cups water

1 large tomato (about 1 cup), diced

2 cups cooked chickpeas, drained and rinsed

2 TB. fresh basil, chopped ₁ tsp.

1½ tsp. fresh oregano leaves, finely chopped, or ½ tsp. dried

¼ tsp. ground black pepper

¼ tsp. sea salt

½ cup whole wheat elbow macaroni

3 TB. plus 1 tsp. Parmesan cheese

1. Heat 4-quart saucepan over medium heat. Place onion, celery, carrot, zucchini, garlic, and olive oil in pot. Cook vegetables for 7 to 8 minutes or until beginning to brown.

2. Add chicken stock, water, tomato, chickpeas, basil, oregano, pepper, and salt. Bring to a boil. Simmer for 10 to 15 minutes.

3. Add whole wheat macaroni and cook for 15 more minutes or until done. Pour in bowls. Immediately before serving sprinkle each bowl with 1 teaspoon Parmesan cheese.

Variation: This soup is so versatile, you can use any cooked vegetables you have on hand. You can also change up the beans. White, red, kidney, or cannellini beans work best.

Chile Corn Chowder

Chowder is a staple in New England, where heavy cream, bacon, and potatoes are typical ingredients. Here poblano peppers give this chowder a southwestern flair while low-fat milk and corn provide the sweetness.

2 cups Roasted Vegetable Stock or Homemade Chicken Stock (see recipe in Chapter 17) or low-sodium canned

1½ cups low-fat milk

1½ cups corn cut off from 3 corn cobs (save cobs), fresh or frozen

¼ cup rice blend or long grain brown rice (uncooked)

2 tsp. olive oil

½ medium onion, small diced (about ½ cup)

1 medium stalk celery, small diced (about ½ cup)

1 medium carrot, small diced (about ½ cup)

½ poblano pepper, seeded and finely chopped

1 garlic clove, peeled and crushed

1 TB. whole wheat flour

½ tsp. ground cumin

1 TB. fresh cilantro leaves, chopped

¼ tsp. sea salt

⅛ tsp. ground black pepper

Yield: 4 servings
Prep time: 10 minutes
Cook time: 35 minutes
Serving size: 1 cup
Each serving has:
178 calories
4 g total fat
1 g saturated fat
6 g protein
31 g carbohydrate
8 g sugars
3 mg cholesterol
4 g fiber
210 mg sodium

1. Heat stock, milk, corn cobs (you may need to cut them in half), and rice blend to a boil in medium saucepan over medium heat, and simmer for 15 minutes. Add corn and cook another 10 minutes. Remove from heat and place in bowl. Set aside.

2. In a large saucepot heat olive oil over medium heat. Mix in onion, celery, carrot, poblano pepper, and garlic. Sauté 3 to 4 minutes covered. Add flour and cook 2 more minutes, stirring frequently.

3. Remove corn cobs from milk mixture. Add milk mixture to vegetable-flour mixture and stir with a wooden spoon. Simmer over medium heat for 8 to 10 minutes. Add cumin, cilantro, salt, and pepper. Cook 5 more minutes. Serve hot.

Variation: This soup is ideal with a cup of cooked shrimp.

Wholesome Habits

Chowders are thick, chunky soups, closer to stews than soups, and usually served with crackers. In New England you can find three types: a tomato-based Manhattan chowder, a cream-based New England chowder, and the third, only found in Rhode Island, is a broth-based Rhode Island chowder.

Hearty Onion Soup

Cubed whole wheat bread tossed with Parmesan cheese make this onion soup a filling and satisfying meal. If you want to impress your family, serve it in individual crocks.

Yield: 5 cups
Prep time: 15 minutes
Cook time: 30 minutes
Serving size: 1 cup
Each serving has:
191 calories
3 g total fat
1 g saturated fat
19 g protein
16 g carbohydrate
4 g sugars
43 mg cholesterol
2 g fiber
105 mg sodium

2 tsp. olive oil

2 large onions, sliced (about 1 lb.)

2 garlic cloves, peeled and crushed

5 cups Homemade Beef Stock (see recipe in Chapter 17) or low-sodium canned beef stock

2 tsp. fresh thyme leaves, chopped

2 bay leaves

4 tsp. red wine

¼ tsp. ground black pepper

2 cups whole wheat bread cut into ½-inch cubes

2 tsp. grated Parmesan

1 tsp. olive oil

1. In a 4-quart saucepot over low heat add olive oil, onion, and garlic; cover pot. Stir occasionally until onion and garlic are caramelized and brown in color, about 20 minutes.

2. Add beef stock, thyme, bay leaves, wine, and black pepper. Bring to boil, then reduce heat, cover, and let simmer on low for 20 to 25 minutes.

3. When soup is almost finished cooking, heat a small sauté pan over high heat. Toss bread with cheese and olive oil in a small bowl. Place bread in hot sauté pan and stir constantly until brown.

4. To assemble, pour 1 cup of soup in each of 5 individual bowls. Evenly divide bread cubes among soup. Serve hot.

 Wholesome Habits

Along with apples and tea, onions are our primary source of quercetin, a potent antioxidant and anti-inflammatory agent believed to decrease the risk for certain cancers.

Part 5

Dinner Designs

Think you'll have to spend hours in the kitchen? Check out our chapter on Dinner in 30 Minutes or Less with meals like Thai Coconut Curry Shrimp with Black Beans or Whole Wheat Pasta with Broccoli. Think you'll have to create elaborate dinners from scratch every night? You'll be thinking differently after you've seen our Double Duty recipes, which help you save time and energy by turning one prep into two meals. For instance, you'll find out how to transform leftovers from Sunday's fabulous Honey-Spiced Chicken into Tuesday's whip-it-up-in-a-flash BBQ Chicken Pizza. Talk about easy!

To accompany these nutritious dinners you'll find a variety of interesting side dishes and starches, many of which could easily stand in for a meal themselves; in addition, we've devoted an entire chapter to flavor-boosting sauces, spice mixes, and condiments—the perfect way to beat the blahs.

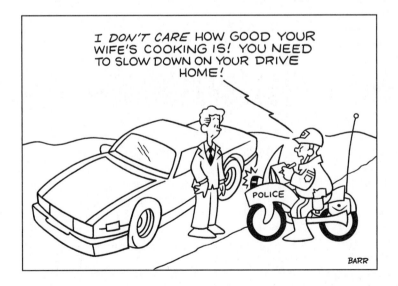

16

Dinner in 30 Minutes or Less

In This Chapter

- ◆ Simply amazing pastas and stir-fries
- ◆ Chicken dinners: more than just broiled breasts
- ◆ Fast, fantastic, and healthy fish finds
- ◆ Pork and beef clean up their act

You don't have to slave over a hot stove to prepare delicious and nutritious clean meals. Nor does eating clean mean you'll have broiled chicken breast and steamed broccoli every night.

In this chapter we show you how to prepare healthy, flavorful meals in 30 minutes or less—meals your family and friends will think you've spent hours preparing (and be amazed by the fact that you didn't). With a well-stocked kitchen it's easy.

In the following recipes all you need is an ample supply of your favorite fresh herbs and spices, an array of colorful accompaniments you can throw in at a moment's notice (we couldn't do without tomatoes, onions, celery, garlic, mangoes, mushrooms, snow peas, sweet potatoes, and carrots), and a stash of quick-cooking proteins like thinly sliced chicken breasts, pork, or beef tenderloin, and lean white fish.

Armed with these ingredients and the recipes in this chapter, you're on your way to enjoying mouth-watering meals like Curried Mango Chicken and Beef Satay in no time at all.

Once you've mastered these recipes, be creative and come up with your own family favorites. Don't feel like making Mussels Italiano? Substitute chicken for the mussels and serve over whole wheat pasta instead. Don't have any broccoli or ground pork for the Whole Wheat Pasta with Broccoli? No problem—try it with zucchini or eggplant and lean ground beef or turkey.

So get out those pots and pans, fire up the oven, and get moving. You don't want to spend all day in the kitchen, do you?

Whole Wheat Pasta with Broccoli

Ground pork and fennel seed add an Italian flair to this ridiculously easy meal, while crushed red pepper gives it a kick.

1 tsp. fennel seed

½ lb. ground pork

1 medium onion, diced

4 garlic cloves, peeled and minced

4 cups Homemade Chicken Stock (see recipe in Chapter 17) or low-sodium canned

1 cup water

1 lb. whole wheat penne pasta

2 bunches broccoli (2½ to 3 lb.), cut into florets

1 cup fresh basil, shredded

4 TB. Pecorino Romano or Parmesan cheese

½ tsp. kosher salt (optional)

¾ tsp. crushed red pepper

Yield: 8 servings
Prep time: 10 minutes
Cook time: 25 minutes
Serving size: 2 cups
Each serving has:
349 calories
10 g total fat
4 g saturated fat
19 g protein
54 g carbohydrate
4 g sugars
25 mg cholesterol
10 g fiber
205 mg sodium

1. Heat a small skillet over medium-high heat. Add fennel and toast, stirring constantly, for 1 to 2 minutes or until fragrant and lightly brown. Let cool for about 1 minute. Crush fennel seed with a mortar and pestle, the back of a metal spoon, or a coffee grinder. Set aside.

2. Spray a large straight-sided skillet with cooking spray and place over medium heat. Add pork, onion, and garlic. Cook until pork is no longer pink and onion and garlic are tender (10 to 15 minutes).

3. When pork is brown, add chicken broth, water, fennel, and uncooked pasta. Cover and bring to a boil. Add more water if necessary. After 5 or 6 minutes, add broccoli, basil, salt (if using), and crushed red pepper flakes. Cook for another 5 to 10 minutes until desired doneness of pasta and broccoli.

4. Serve in large bowls. Right before serving sprinkle each serving with ½ tablespoon grated Pecorino Romano or Parmesan.

Variation: For a summery version of this dish, replace the broccoli with 4 cups roasted eggplant (about 4 small or 2 large eggplants) and 2 medium tomatoes, seeded and diced. To roast eggplant, heat oven to 425°F, peel eggplant and cut into ¹/₂-inch thick slices. Line a sheet pan with aluminum foil and spray with cooking spray. Place eggplant on pan and spray eggplant with cooking spray. Bake eggplant in oven for 15 minutes, turning once after 8 minutes. When cool enough to handle, cut eggplant into cubes.

Clean Cuts _____

You can substitute the ground pork and fennel with,
6 ounces fresh pork sausage with casings removed (break
the meat up into small pieces before cooking). Avoid store-
bought brands of sausage, which are typically high in fat and
sodium and often contain artificial colors, preservatives, and
additives. Instead, find a butcher who makes his own sausage
fresh using his own spice mix. Some butchers use prepackaged
spice mixes, which are unlikely to be clean. Ask before you
buy.

Mediterranean Carrot Stir-Fry

Winter vegetables are given a Mediterranean treatment when they're sprinkled with a *gremolata*-type mixture of chopped parsley, orange zest, garlic, and olive oil in this vegetarian entrée. It's served on a bed of whole wheat couscous blended with kasha (buckwheat groats) for a nutty texture and taste.

1½ tsp. olive oil

1 lb. carrots, peeled and sliced into ¼-inch pieces

1 parsnip (5 to 6 oz.), peeled and sliced into ¼-inch slices

1 medium onion, thinly sliced

¼ head of cabbage (8 or 9 oz.), thinly sliced

½ tsp. kosher salt

¼ tsp. coriander seeds, crushed

⅛ tsp. ground black pepper

¼ cup orange juice

½ plus ⅓ cup water

¼ cup whole grain kasha (buckwheat groats)

⅓ cup whole wheat couscous

2 TB. fresh parsley, finely chopped

1 garlic clove, peeled and crushed

1 tsp. grated orange or lemon zest or ½ tsp. orange zest and ½ tsp. lemon zest

Yield: 4 servings
Prep time: 10 minutes
Cook time: 20 minutes
Serving size: 1 cup vegetables, ⅔ cup grain mixture
Each serving has:
253 calories
3 g total fat
0 g saturated fat
7 g protein
53 g carbohydrate
11 g sugars
0 mg cholesterol
11 g fiber
338 mg sodium

1. Heat 1 teaspoon olive oil in a large skillet over medium heat. Add carrots, parsnip, onion, and cabbage. Cover and cook for 10 minutes. Mix in salt, coriander, black pepper, and orange juice. Cover and cook for another 10 minutes. If mixture begins to stick to pan, add water, as needed, one tablespoon at a time.

2. While vegetables are cooking, bring ½ cup water to a boil in a small saucepan. Add kasha, stir, cover, and reduce heat to simmer. Cook for 10 minutes. In another small saucepan, bring ⅓ cup water to a boil. Remove from heat, add couscous, and cover tightly. Let sit for 7 to 8 minutes. When both grains are cooked, blend together in small bowl, add a pinch of salt, and set aside.

3. On clean cutting board, blend finely chopped parsley with crushed garlic, orange zest, and remaining ½ teaspoon olive oil to form a crumbly paste.

4. To assemble, in individual bowls place ⅔ cup grain mixture, top with 1 cup vegetables, and sprinkle with 1½ teaspoons parsley mixture. Serve.

Variation: If you're looking for more protein, try adding a cup of cooked chicken or pork to this meal. Still want to keep it vegetarian? Opt for 1 cup diced firm tofu.

 Clean Meanings

Gremolata is an Italian condiment made with fresh parsley, garlic, and lemon or orange. It's traditionally served as a topping for osso buco (braised veal shanks).

Tofu-Pineapple-Broccoli Stir-Fry

Tofu takes on the flavor of whatever food you pair it with. Here it's tossed with Homemade Hoisin Sauce, garlic, broccoli, and pineapple for an Asian-inspired dish. Cooking the brown rice ahead of time makes this dish a snap to prepare.

Yield: 4 or 5 servings
Prep time: 15 minutes
Cook time: 10 minutes
Serving size: 1 cup tofu-vegetable mixture and ½ cup cooked brown rice
Each serving has:
266 calories
8 g total fat
1 g saturated fat
12 g protein
38 g carbohydrate
9 g sugars
0 mg cholesterol
6 g fiber
169 mg sodium

1 tsp. canola or peanut oil

5 cups Chinese broccoli, coarsely chopped

½ medium onion, sliced

3 garlic cloves, peeled and minced

½ large red bell pepper, seeds and ribs removed, sliced

16 oz. tofu, firm or extra firm, diced

¾ cup pineapple, diced

2½ TB. Homemade Hoisin Sauce (see recipe in Chapter 21)

½ tsp. crushed red pepper (optional)

2½ cups cooked brown rice

5 tsp. unsalted peanuts, finely chopped (optional)

1. Heat oil in a large wok or sauté pan over high heat. Add broccoli, onion, garlic, and red bell pepper. Stir quickly for about 5 minutes.

2. Add tofu, pineapple, and Homemade Hoisin Sauce. Cook for another 4 or 5 minutes. Sprinkle with crushed red pepper (if using).

3. To assemble, spoon ½ cup brown rice in each bowl, top with 1 cup tofu-vegetable mixture, and sprinkle 1 teaspoon chopped peanuts over the top. Serve immediately.

Wholesome Habits

Chinese broccoli, known as Gai Lan and Chinese kale, has long dark green leaves, small florets, and long green stems. It is milder and sweeter than regular broccoli. Broccolini is a cross between regular broccoli and Gai Lan. If you can't find Chinese broccoli, you can substitute broccoli rabe (also called rapini), broccolini, or regular broccoli instead.

Curried Mango Chicken with Quinoa

Aromatic spices mingle with sweet mango, toasted almonds, and nutty quinoa to give this surprisingly easy weeknight chicken dinner an exotic appeal.

1 tsp. curry powder

1 tsp. ground cumin

1 tsp. fresh ginger, finely minced

1 garlic clove, peeled and crushed

½ tsp. salt

12 oz. boneless, skinless chicken breast, cut into bite-sized pieces (about 1 to 2 chicken breasts)

¼ cup slivered almonds

1 tsp. olive oil

1 medium onion, chopped

1½ cup quinoa

1 cup Homemade Chicken Stock (see recipe in Chapter 17) or low-sodium canned

2 cups water

1½ cups cooked chickpeas, drained and rinsed

1 large mango, peeled and chopped into bite-sized pieces (about 2 cups)

1 cup fresh parsley, chopped (about one bunch)

Yield: 6 servings
Prep time: 10 minutes
Cook time: 20 minutes
Serving size: 1 cup
Each serving has:
403 calories
10 g total fat
1 g saturated fat
30 g protein
49 g carbohydrate
9 g sugars
48 g cholesterol
8 g fiber
342 mg sodium

1. In a small bowl mix curry, cumin, ginger, garlic, and ¼ teaspoon salt to make a spice blend. Place chicken in a small bowl, sprinkle with 2 teaspoons spice blend, and mix.

2. Toast almonds in small dry sauté pan over high heat for 1 or 2 minutes or until lightly brown. Remove from heat and set aside.

3. In large saucepan, heat olive oil over medium heat. Add chicken to skillet and cook 5 or 6 minutes or until no longer pink in center. Remove chicken from skillet and cover to keep warm.

4. Add onion to saucepan, stirring frequently until soft, about 3 minutes. Add quinoa, cooking for about 1 or 2 minutes more until slightly brown. Stir in chicken stock, water, remaining ¼ teaspoon salt, and remaining spice mixture. Cover and simmer over medium-high heat for 15 minutes.

5. Add cooked chicken, chickpeas, and mango. Cover and heat through, about 5 to 10 more minutes. Sprinkle with toasted almonds and parsley and serve immediately.

Clean Cuts

Mangoes are available fresh or frozen. The advantage of buying frozen is that the mango can be used the same day. Most fresh store-bought mangoes need to ripen for at least a few days before they are ready to be eaten. You'll know a mango is ripe because it smells fragrant and is soft enough to leave an indent when pressed.

Lemon Chicken with Minty Peas and Carrots

This recipe calls to mind the bright taste of summer. Broiled chicken breast is doused with a light lemon broth then topped with a dollop or two of Minty Pea and Carrot Purée.

Yield: 4 servings

Prep time: 10 minutes, plus 10 minutes to prepare Minty Pea and Carrot Purée

Cook time: 10 minutes

Serving size: 3 ounces chicken breast, ¼ cup lemon broth, and 2 tablespoons pea and carrot purée

---

Each serving has:

329 calories

13 g total fat

3 g saturated fat

41 g protein

52 g carbohydrate

1 g sugars

52 mg cholesterol

1 g fiber

451 mg sodium

---

12 oz. boneless, skinless chicken breast, cut into 4 cutlets (1–2 chicken breasts)

1 cup Homemade Chicken Stock (see recipe in Chapter 17) or low-sodium canned

2 tsp. lemon zest

Juice of 1 lemon (2–3 tsp.)

8 TB. Minty Pea and Carrot Purée (see recipe in Chapter 21)

1. Heat oven to 425°F. Place chicken cutlets on cookie sheet sprayed with cooking spray or dry stoneware. Bake for 10 minutes.

2. In small saucepot, heat chicken broth, lemon juice, and zest until almost boiling.

3. To assemble, place one chicken breast cutlet in a bowl, ladle ¼ cup lemon chicken broth over top, and finish with 2 tablespoons pea and carrot purée, brought to room temperature. Serve immediately.

Dirty Secrets _____

Some conventionally grown lemons have a wax coating to protect them during shipping, so if you plan on using the peel for zest, be sure and buy wax-free organically-grown lemons and limes.

Catfish with Roasted Sweet Potato Hash

Catfish pairs beautifully with roasted sweet potato and edamame—a fresh soybean that looks like a lima bean, but has a sweeter taste.

3 cups sweet potato, peeled and cut into ¾-inch dice

2 garlic cloves, peeled and minced

½ medium onion, chopped

½ tsp. sea salt

¼ tsp. cracked black pepper

1½ cups shelled edamame

1 TB. maple syrup

1 lb. catfish fillets, cut into 4-oz. pieces

½ tsp. fresh thyme leaves or ⅛ tsp. dried

¼ tsp. cayenne

Yield: 4 servings
Prep time: 10 minutes
Cook time: 30 minutes
Serving size: 1 cup vegetables, 4 ounces catfish
Each serving has:
316 calories
11 g total fat
2 g saturated fat
24 g protein
32 g carbohydrate
10 g sugars
53 mg cholesterol
6 g fiber
412 mg sodium

1. Preheat oven to 425°F. Spray a 9×13-inch roasting pan with cooking spray. Toss sweet potato, garlic, and onion in pan. Spray with cooking spray. Sprinkle with ¼ teaspoon sea salt and cracked black pepper, cover with aluminum foil, and bake for 20 minutes.

2. While sweet potatoes are cooking, cook edamame according to package directions, omitting salt. Drain and set aside.

3. When sweet potatoes are done, take out of the oven and turn heat up to high broil. Sprinkle catfish with remaining ¼ teaspoon sea salt, thyme, and cayenne. Add edamame and maple syrup to cooked sweet potatoes in pan. Mix with a metal spatula. Move vegetables to side of pan and place catfish on the empty side of the pan. Spray catfish with cooking spray.

4. Put catfish and sweet potatoes in oven, uncovered, for 7 to 10 minutes or until catfish is white and flakes easily with fork. To serve place 4 ounces of catfish on a plate and top with 1 cup vegetables. Serve immediately.

Variation: Any mild white fish or shellfish can be substituted for catfish. Try tilapia, shrimp, sole, or hake.

Wholesome Habits

Sweet potatoes are brimming with vitamin A. One medium baked sweet potato contains more than four times the recommended daily intake for this nutrient. Sweet potatoes are also high in fiber, vitamin C, potassium, and manganese.

Thai Coconut Curry Shrimp with Black Beans

Low-fat coconut milk and spicy *green curry* paste combine with shrimp, bok choy, and black beans to bring the flavors of Thailand to your door.

Yield: 4 servings
Prep time: 10 minutes
Cook time: 10 minutes
Serving size: 1 cup
Each serving has:
203 calories
6 g total fat
3 g saturated fat
22 g protein
15 g carbohydrate
2 g sugars
128 mg cholesterol
5 g fiber
241 mg sodium

¾ **cup low-fat coconut milk**

¼ **cup water**

2 tsp. lime juice

1 tsp. sesame seed oil

⅓ **cup sweet red bell pepper, chopped**

2 garlic cloves, peeled and minced

½ **small onion, chopped**

¾ **lb. raw shrimp (about 20 shrimp), peeled with tail off**

2 cups bok choy, sliced

2 tsp. green curry paste

¼ **cup fresh Thai basil or cilantro leaves, shredded**

1 cup cooked black beans, drained and rinsed

1. In small bowl, mix coconut milk, water, and lime juice. Set aside.

2. Heat sesame seed oil in large wok or skillet over medium-high heat. Place red pepper, garlic, and onion in wok or skillet and sauté for 1 or 2 minutes, stirring frequently. Add shrimp, bok choy, curry paste, and Thai basil. Cook for 1 to 2 minutes until shrimp turns white. Add black beans and coconut mixture. Heat through for another minute.

3. Serve with cooked brown rice or Pineapple Brown Rice (see recipe in Chapter 20).

Variation: If you like mollusks, try replacing the shrimp with about 50 little neck clams. Their sweet-salty taste pairs beautifully with the black beans, curry, and coconut milk.

 Clean Meanings

Green curry is a mixture of many different spices. It typically includes green chiles, onion, lime, coriander, lemongrass, soy sauce, garlic, and ginger. Although recipes vary, it is usually hot and spicy. It is a common ingredient in Thai cuisine.

Mussels Italiano

This classic Italian dish is full of flavor, with the garlic, onions, basil, and tomatoes complementing the briny broth produced by the mussels. You'll want to sop up every drop.

2 lb. mussels, rinsed and cleaned

2 tsp. extra-virgin olive oil

3 large garlic cloves, peeled and minced

¼ cup medium onion, chopped

3 TB. fresh basil, chopped (about 8 leaves)

4 medium tomatoes (about 1 lb.), seeded and coarsely chopped

¼ cup white wine

¼ tsp. ground black pepper

Yield: 6 servings
Prep time: 5 minutes
Cook time: 10 minutes
Serving size: 8 to 10 mussels per person
Each serving has:
177 calories
5 g total fat
1 g saturated fat
19 g protein
10 g carbohydrate
2 g sugars
42 mg cholesterol
1 g fiber
433 mg sodium

1. Clean mussels by rinsing them under cold running water and brushing them with a stiff kitchen brush. Pull out the beard, (the fuzzy hairs sticking out of the side of the mussel), by giving it a yank. (You can also buy beardless mussels.) Remove any dead ones (shells that are opened or cracked).

2. Heat olive oil in a large 8-quart pot over medium-high heat. Add garlic, onion, and basil. Cook for about 1 minute, or until soft. Mix in tomatoes, wine, and black pepper, then heat for another 2 minutes. Add mussels, bring to a boil, and cover. Cook for about 4 minutes or until mussels open. Serve immediately in big bowls.

Tip: Serve these mussels with pasta or rice, or make whole wheat garlic bread. To make garlic bread, heat oven to 425°F. Thinly slice a loaf of Italian whole wheat bread, and top each slice with ¼ teaspoon extra-virgin olive oil mixed with ⅛ teaspoon minced garlic and 2 slivers of fresh basil leaf, and sprinkle with ½ teaspoon low-fat mozzarella. Toast in oven for about 1 minute or until edges begin to brown. Three slices per serving.

Clean Cuts

Most mussels are now cultivated through aquaculture, making them much cleaner (less likely to have seabed mud and grit in them) than their wild counterparts. If you're going to keep them overnight or even for a couple of days, store them in a bowl in the refrigerator covered with a wet towel. Don't store in plain water, as it will kill them.

Beef Satay on Rice Noodles

Everyone loves beef on a stick. Here skewered beef is served on a bed of rice noodles with snow peas and shredded carrots. The dressing highlights Asian flavors of hoisin, lime, and finished with peanuts.

Yield: 6 servings
Prep time: 10 minutes
Cook time: 15 minutes
Serving size: 2 beef skewers, 1 cup rice noodles, and 1 cup vegetables
Each serving has:
374 calories
12 g total fat
2 g saturated fat
18 g protein
48 g carbohydrate
10 g sugars
34 mg cholesterol
4 g fiber
212 mg sodium

Wholesome Habits

Thanks to the abundant amount of snow peas and carrots, one serving of this dish provides more than 100 percent of the recommended daily value of vitamins A and C and nearly 60 percent of the recommended daily value of vitamin K.

1½ cups fresh cilantro leaves

9 green onions, both green and white parts chopped

3 tsp. fresh ginger, chopped

2 TB. sesame seed oil

2 TB. Homemade Hoisin Sauce (see recipe in Chapter 21)

2 TB. water

¾ cup fresh orange juice

1 tsp. jalapeño pepper, finely chopped (about ¼ pepper)

12 oz. beef tenderloin or strip steak, cut into 1-oz. strips

12 wooden or metal skewers

3 medium carrots, peeled and shredded (about 3 cups)

12 oz. snow peas (about 4 cups)

1 (8-oz.) package thin rice noodle sticks

4 TB. unsalted, roasted peanuts, chopped

1. Fill a 4-quart pot with water and bring to a boil over high heat. Place cilantro, green onions, ginger, sesame seed oil, hoisin sauce, water, orange juice, and jalapeño pepper in the bowl of a food processor. Process on high for about 30 seconds. Scrape down the sides of the bowl with a rubber spatula and process again for another 30 seconds until smooth. Place 1 tablespoon of dressing in separate bowl and set the rest aside.

2. Heat oven to high broil. Thread each beef strip on a metal skewer. Brush skewered beef with reserved tablespoon dressing, discarding any leftover dressing. Place beef on cookie sheet or stoneware and broil on high for 2 minutes. Turn meat over and broil 2 more minutes.

3. While meat is cooking, put rice noodles in boiling water. Cook for 2 minutes. Remove noodles from pot, but keep water boiling. Then drop in snow peas and shredded carrot, cooking for another minute. Drain.

4. To assemble, evenly divide noodles, snow peas, and carrots among 6 bowls. Top each with 2 beef skewers, 2 tablespoons dressing, and 2 teaspoons chopped peanuts. Serve immediately.

Steak Diane

Steak Diane is typically doused in butter and cream. This light version uses beef stock and a smidgen of soymilk instead, along with mushrooms, onions, red wine, and fresh herbs. It's an ideal dish to serve for a romantic dinner.

4 (4-oz.) beef tenderloin steaks, trimmed of all fat

¼ tsp. sea salt

⅛ tsp. ground black pepper

1 tsp. extra-virgin olive oil

1 garlic clove, peeled and minced

2 TB. onion, chopped

1 (8-oz.) package whole white mushrooms, coarsely chopped

¼ cup red table wine

1 tsp. fresh thyme leaves, chopped or ¼ tsp. dried

2 TB. unsweetened soymilk or 1 percent low-fat milk

1 cup Homemade Beef Stock (see recipe in Chapter 17) or low-sodium canned

Yield: 4 servings
Prep time: 15 minutes
Cook time: 10 minutes
Serving size: one steak and about ¼ cup mushrooms
Each serving has:
277 calories
9 g total fat
3 g saturated fat
38 g protein
4 g carbohydrate
1 g sugars
84 mg cholesterol
1 g fiber
227 mg sodium

1. Sprinkle both sides of meat with sea salt and black pepper. Heat a large skillet over medium-high heat. Add olive oil and cook beef tenderloin for 2 minutes on each side. Remove from pan, place on plate. Cover to keep warm and set aside.

2. Add garlic, onion, and mushrooms to pan. Sauté for about 3 minutes. Then add wine, thyme, and soymilk.

3. Reduce the heat to medium-low and place the steaks back into the pan with mushrooms. Pour in any juice. Cook about 2 more minutes and serve immediately. Serve over All-Purpose Multigrain Blend or brown rice or paired with Veggie Maple Mashed Potatoes (see recipes in Chapter 20).

Wholesome Habits

Steak Diane was originally created in the 1920s when tableside flambé cooking was all the rage. It was named after the Greek goddess of the hunt, Diana, and was prepared with venison.

Sweet n' Sauerkraut Pork

In this German-inspired dish, pork tenderloin is nestled on a bed of cabbage, onions, apples, and sauerkraut. Slow-cooking these ingredients produce a combination of flavors that is mildly sweet, salty, sour, and savory.

Yield: 4 servings
Prep time: 10 minutes
Cook time: 25 minutes
Serving size: 4 ounces pork tenderloin, 1 cup vegetables
Each serving has:
231 calories
5 g total fat
1 g saturated fat
31 g protein
16 g carbohydrate
10 g sugars
82 mg cholesterol
4 g fiber
199 mg sodium

16 oz. pork tenderloin, cut into 4 (4-oz.) cutlets

⅛ tsp. paprika

⅛ tsp. ground black pepper

⅛ tsp. ground coriander

½ tsp. olive oil

1 medium onion (about ½ cup), thinly sliced

4 cups thinly sliced cabbage (about ¼ head)

¼ cup apple juice, unsweetened

¾ cup water

2 small apples, peeled, cored, and diced (about 2 cups)

1 cup all-natural, low-sodium sauerkraut

1 cup fresh parsley, finely chopped

1. Sprinkle both sides of meat with paprika, black pepper, and coriander. Spray large skillet with cooking spray and heat over medium-high heat, then place pork tenderloins in pan. Cook for 2 minutes on each side. Remove meat from pan, place on plate, cover, and set aside.

2. Lower the heat to medium-low and add olive oil to the same skillet. Add onions and cabbage. Cover and cook, stirring occasionally, for about 10 minutes. Add apple juice, water, and diced apples. Cover and cook another 5 to 10 minutes. Mix in sauerkraut, then put pork back in. Cover and cook through another 5 to 8 minutes. Sprinkle with chopped parsley and cover for about a minute. Serve hot.

> **Clean Cuts**
>
> Sauerkraut is fermented cabbage. Many canned or packaged versions have added salt along with other unclean ingredients like sugar and preservatives. Look for all-natural, low-sodium brands of sauerkraut, which contain simply cabbage and water (no added salt). Sodium levels for these clean versions run around a reasonable 200 to 250 milligrams per ½ cup.

Chapter 17

Weekend Warriors: Big Batch Cooking

In This Chapter

◆ Making basic stocks and sauces

◆ Baking pizza dough and flatbreads

◆ Creating Sunday dinners any day of the week

Certainly quick cooking meals are essential to surviving in our fast-paced world, but there are times when we seek solace in a slow-cooked meal—in the aroma of a perfectly cooked roast beef, the bubbles of a gently simmering stew, or the yeasty rise of baked bread. These are the kinds of home-cooked comfort foods that thrive on long, slow cooking times.

This chapter is dedicated to preparing the types of food your grandmother might have made—long, slow, and involved—and the kind of food many people crave, but don't often make.

What makes these recipes so special? Because they are made from scratch using fresh vegetables, beans, grains, and meats, cleaning up these old-fashioned meals in order to reduce the fat, sodium, and calories is surprisingly easy.

In addition, spending more time cooking big batches translates into less time in the kitchen later on. For example, if you make a double batch of Orange Beef Stew or Thanksgiving Meatloaf, you'll have enough for lunch a few days later. Or you can freeze individual portions for a quick "frozen" dinner you can microwave.

Making your own stocks and sauces are another important part of eating clean. They taste better than canned, and they are also healthier, as they do not rely on salt, sugar, or additives like MSG to provide flavor. Surprisingly easy to make, they can save you money, too.

Instead of throwing out wilted or past-their-prime vegetables, toss them into a stock. Have left over chicken, turkey, or beef bones from dinner? Why not whip up a quick stock? Although we always start with raw, uncooked chicken, turkey, or beef bones in our recipes, it is possible to make a perfectly good stock using precooked (after the meat has been removed) chicken, turkey, or beef bones.

You'll find these clean comfort foods healing for the body as well as the soul. Make them as your own grandmother would, with tender love and care, and you'll never go wrong.

Basic Tomato Sauce

Roasting tomatoes brings out their sweetness, so you don't need to add much sugar to this chunky tomato sauce flecked with green basil and parsley. Limiting the sugar also allows the fresh, clean taste of the herbs and vegetables to shine through.

4 lb. fresh plum tomatoes, cored and cut into 1½-inch pieces

4 tsp. olive oil

½ medium onion, finely chopped

4 garlic cloves, peeled and minced

2 tsp. fresh basil, finely chopped

2 tsp. fresh parsley, finely chopped

1 tsp. Sucanat

1 tsp. kosher salt

¼ tsp. ground black pepper

Yield: 10 servings (5 cups)
Prep time: 15 minutes
Cook time: 70 minutes
Serving size: ½ cup
Each serving has:
55 calories
2 g total fat
0 g saturated fat
2 g protein
9 g carbohydrate
5 g sugars
0 mg cholesterol
2 g fiber
106 mg sodium

1. Heat oven to 425°F. Place tomatoes in an 8×11-inch roasting pan. Coat tomatoes with 2 teaspoons of olive oil. Roast for 45 minutes.

2. When done, put tomatoes in the bowl of a food processor and process until smooth (about 1 or 2 minutes) in two batches. Strain sauce through a sieve, pressing down with the back of wooden spoon. Seeds and skin will be left behind, while pulp will go through. (Make sure the holes of the strainer are not so big that the seeds can pass through but are large enough to let pulp through.)

3. Heat remaining olive oil in a 4-quart saucepot over medium heat. Add onion and garlic and sauté for about 3 minutes, until onion softens and turns translucent. Add puréed tomatoes, basil, parsley, Sucanat, salt, and pepper. Bring to a slow boil over medium-high heat. Reduce heat to low, cover, and simmer for 20 minutes. Serve immediately over pasta or cool in individual containers and store in the refrigerator or freezer.

Clean Cuts

Compared to fresh, cooked tomatoes have higher levels of lycopene (the chemical responsible for tomato's red color), an antioxidant that is believed to reduce the risk of heart disease and certain cancers.

Homemade Chicken Stock

Once you make your own chicken stock you'll never go back to canned. It has an intense, chicken flavor even without the salt. Make a double batch so you always have some on hand.

Yield: 8 cups
Prep time: 20 minutes
Cook time: 1 hour
Serving size: ½ cup
Each serving has:
20 calories
0 g total fat
0 g saturated fat
4 g protein
0 g carbohydrate
0 g sugars
9 mg cholesterol
0 g fiber
13 mg sodium

1 lb. chicken bones (about 6 lb. split chicken breast, with skin and breast meat removed)

10 cups water

1 medium onion, coarsely chopped

2 medium carrots, peeled and chopped

1 large stalk celery, coarsely chopped

½ cup fresh parsley leaves

8 whole black peppercorns

3 bay leaves

6 sprigs thyme

1. If using chicken breasts, skin and debone (you can have your butcher do this for you) the breasts. Wrap and refrigerate or freeze boneless chicken breasts in sealed freezer bag for another time.

2. Heat water in an 8-quart stockpot over medium-high heat. Add chicken bones, vegetables, parsley, peppercorns, bay leaves, and thyme. Bring to a boil. Reduce heat to low, partially cover, and let simmer for 40 minutes.

3. Set a strainer over a large bowl and pour stock through strainer. Discard chicken bones, cooked vegetables, and spices. You should have a nice, rich, chicken stock. Transfer into shallow bowls. Cool for about 15 minutes inside an ice water bath in a large pan. When cool, store in refrigerator. Chill overnight.

4. The next day, skim off any fat that has solidified on the top of the stock. This ensures your chicken stock will be fat-free (or close to it). Store in tightly covered containers in refrigerator or freezer.

Variation: Try using turkey bones instead of chicken.

Clean Cuts

If you don't like handling raw chicken or turkey bones, you can use cooked. In this recipe replace the raw chicken bones with about 2 pounds of cooked turkey breast bone from the Roast Turkey Breast with Lemon and Oregano recipe later in this chapter. Then follow the same directions. You can also use the same amount of cooked chicken bones.

Homemade Beef Stock

Taking the extra step to roast the bones gives this stock its dark caramel color and rich meaty taste. If you're having trouble finding beef bones for soup stock just ask your butcher.

Yield: 12 cups
Prep time: 5 minutes
Cook time: 4½ hours
Serving size: ½ cup
Each serving has:
39 calories
0 g total fat
0 g saturated fat
8 g protein
1 g carbohydrate
0 g sugars
21 mg cholesterol
0 g fiber
19 mg sodium

6 lb. beef bones, cut into 4 or 5-inch pieces (ask your butcher to do this)

2 medium onions, coarsely chopped

1 large stalk celery, coarsely chopped

2 medium carrots, peeled and coarsely chopped

2 garlic cloves, peeled and cut in half

1 gallon water

3 bay leaves

1 tsp. black peppercorns

6 sprigs thyme

1. Heat oven to 450°F. Place beef bones in large roasting pan along with onions, celery, carrots, and garlic. Roast in oven for 1½ hours until well-browned. Drain off excess oils.

2. Place cooked bones and vegetables in an 8-quart stockpot and cover with water. Add bay leaves, peppercorns, and thyme. Bring to a boil over medium-high heat then reduce to a simmer. Cook partially covered for 3½ hours, stirring occasionally.

3. Set a strainer over a large bowl or pot and pour stock through strainer. Discard beef bones, cooked vegetables, bay leaves, and spices. You should have a dark, rich, beef stock. Transfer into shallow bowls. Cool for about 15 minutes in an ice water bath in a large pan, then store cooled stock in refrigerator. Chill overnight.

4. The next day, skim off any fat that has solidified on the top of the stock. This ensures your beef stock will be fat-free (or close to it). Store in a tightly covered container in the refrigerator or freezer.

Clean Cuts

You can make this stock with any type of meat bones, including veal or pork. And if you don't have raw bones, you can use precooked bones. You still roast them until they're brown, it just won't take as long to do so (depending on the type of bone, 30 to 45 minutes would probably be enough).

Roasted Vegetable Stock

You don't have to have perfect vegetables to make this vegetable stock. This recipe calls for the most common—celery, carrots, onions, and tomato—but feel free to throw in asparagus, mushrooms, green beans, or any other vegetable. Just be careful not to add too many strong flavored vegetables, such as parsnips or turnips, as their flavor can overpower the stock. Roasting brings out the natural sweetness of the vegetables.

2 medium carrots, peeled and coarsely chopped

2 medium onions, peeled and coarsely chopped

1 large stalk celery, coarsely chopped

2 garlic cloves, peeled and sliced in half

1 medium tomato, cut into 1-inch pieces

4 sprigs thyme

2 bay leaves

½ tsp. black peppercorns

1 tsp. olive oil

4 cups water

Yield: 3 cups
Prep time: 10 minutes
Cook time: 1½ hours
Serving size: ½ cup
Each serving has:
11 calories
0 g total fat
0 g saturated fat
0 g protein
2 g carbohydrate
1 g sugars
0 mg cholesterol
1 g fiber
8 mg sodium

1. Heat oven to 425°F. Place carrots, onions, celery, garlic, and tomatoes in large roasting pan. Coat vegetables with olive oil. Roast in oven for about 50 minutes, or until vegetables are a nice dark brown color.

2. Remove vegetables from oven, then pour 2 cups water into pan, scraping up caramelized bits from bottom and sides. Pour vegetables, vegetable mixture, and remaining 2 cups water, bay leaves, peppercorns, and thyme into an 8-quart stockpot and bring to a boil over medium-high heat. Reduce heat to a simmer, partially cover, and cook for 30 minutes.

3. Set a strainer over a large bowl and pour stock through the strainer. Discard cooked vegetables, bay leaves, and spices. You should have a dark, rich, vegetable stock. Transfer into shallow bowls. Cool for about 15 minutes in an ice water bath in a large pan. Store stock in refrigerator or freeze until ready to use.

Wholesome Habits

All vegetables are good for you, but some rank higher on the nutritional scale than others. For instance kale, spinach, collard greens, and other leafy greens stand head and shoulders above the rest. Next come pumpkin, sweet potato, carrots, and broccoli. To find out more about where vegetables fall on the nutritional scale and why, check out the Center for Science in the Public Interest report called *Veggie vs. Veggie: Rating Rutabagas* at http://cspinet.org/nah/archives.html (it's in the Archives, under January/February 2009).

White Beans with Rosemary

Mild tasting white beans cook up creamy and delicious with a hint of rosemary and some garlic. You can eat them plain as a side dish with a sprinkle of lemon and a drizzle of olive oil or you can use them in soups, salads, stews, and casseroles.

1 lb. northern white beans, dry (2½ cups)

4 garlic cloves, peeled and sliced

3 bay leaves

8 rosemary stems or 6 tarragon stems or any other fresh whole leaf herb

1 tsp. sea salt

¼ tsp. cracked black pepper

Yield: 14 servings
Prep time: 5 minutes, plus an overnight soak
Cook time: 1 hour
Serving size: ½ cup
Each serving has:
110 calories
0 g total fat
0 g saturated fat
7 g protein
20 g carbohydrate
1 g sugars
0 mg cholesterol
6 g fiber
88 mg sodium

1. Clean and sort beans, picking out any rocks or dirt. Place in a 4-quart saucepot with 5 cups water. Soak overnight.

2. Drain soaked beans in colander. Put 4 cups fresh water in the pot, along with beans, garlic, and bay leaves. Heat over medium-high heat until beans come to a gentle boil. Lower the heat to simmer and partially cover. Cook for 1 hour, stirring occasionally.

3. After beans cook for 1 hour, add rosemary, salt, and pepper. Cook another 20 to 30 minutes until beans are tender. Serve hot or store in the refrigerator.

Variations: You can cook almost any type of dried bean this way. Try red beans, kidney beans, navy beans, lima beans, cannellini beans, or chickpeas. Cooking times may vary depending on the size of the bean, so be sure and read the package directions first.

Wholesome Habits

Forgot to soak your beans overnight? No problem. Do this instead: Pour beans in saucepot with enough water to cover. Heat on high until beans come to a gentle boil (beans will start to float to the top). Boil for 2 minutes. Take off the heat, cover, and let beans soak in water for 2 to 3 hours (the longer they soak the less time they will need to cook). Then cook as you would normally.

Whole Wheat Pizza Dough

Making your own pizza dough isn't as hard as some people think. This one has a robust wheaty flavor and a crisp, crunchy texture, plus it's low in sodium.

Yield: 1 large pizza *(12 slices)*
Prep time: 20 minutes
Cook time: 40 minutes
Serving size: 1 slice
Each serving has:
165 calories
4 g total fat
0 g saturated fat
5 g protein
29 g carbohydrate
2 g sugars
0 g cholesterol
5 g fiber
99 mg sodium

2½ tsp. active dry yeast (1 package is about 2¼ tsp.)

1 cup plus 2 TB. warm water (100–110°F)

2 TB. Sucanat

3 TB. canola oil

2 TB. pineapple or orange juice

3 to 4 cups of whole wheat flour

½ cup spelt flour

½ tsp. sea salt

1. Combine yeast, warm water, Sucanat, and oil in a large bowl and let sit about 5 minutes, until yeast begins to bubble.

2. Add pineapple juice, 3½ cups whole wheat flour, spelt flour, and salt. Stir until a soft dough forms. Dough will be slightly sticky; add more whole wheat flour as necessary. Turn dough onto lightly floured surface and knead until smooth and elastic, about 5 to 10 minutes.

3. Place dough in a greased bowl (either sprayed with cooking spray or lightly oiled). Let rise for 1 hour. Punch down dough and roll out into pizza.

Variation: This recipe is great for making flatbread. Simply divide the pizza dough in half, then form into a 10×10-inch square on a pan sprayed with cooking spray or a baking stone. Heat oven to 450°F and brush dough with 2 teaspoons olive oil mixed with 1 teaspoon Parmesan cheese. Bake for 10 to 12 minutes. Add caramelized onions for more great flavor.

 Clean Cuts

The best way to measure flour is to gently scoop it into a 1 cup measure and level it off with the back of a knife.

Steamed Pork Buns

Make these homey steamed pork buns when you want a special treat. Their exotic flavor comes from the combination of fragrant Chinese five-spice powder and homemade *hoisin sauce*. Napa cabbage and celery add crunch as well as fiber.

1 lb. pork tenderloin steak

½ tsp. Chinese five-spice powder

½ cup sliced green onions

1 medium stalk celery, finely diced

2 cups napa cabbage, finely sliced, plus 3 or 4 uncut leaves for steaming

6 TB. Homemade Hoisin Sauce (see recipe in Chapter 21)

2 TB. honey

1½ tsp. fresh ginger, minced

2 garlic cloves, peeled and minced

1 recipe Whole Wheat Pizza Dough (see recipe earlier in this chapter)

1½ tsp. baking powder

Yield: 10 pork buns
Prep time: 20 minutes
Cook time: 2 hours
Serving size: 1 steamed pork bun
Each serving has:
284 calories
7 g total fat
1 g saturated fat
16 g protein
41 g carbohydrate
8 g sugars
29 mg cholesterol
6 g fiber
244 mg sodium

1. Heat oven to 300°F. Sprinkle pork tenderloin with five-spice powder and rub spice into meat. Place meat in a small roasting pan, cover with aluminum foil, and cook for 1½ hours.

2. While meat is cooking make pizza dough. In a medium bowl, mix together green onions, celery, cabbage, hoisin sauce, honey, ginger, and garlic.

3. Remove meat from oven, uncover, and let cool for about 10 minutes. Shred with a fork and toss with vegetable mixture.

4. After pizza dough has risen, punch down and knead in baking powder until well incorporated. Let dough rest for 5 minutes.

5. Fill an 8-quart pot ¼ full with water. Place over medium-high heat and bring to a boil.

6. Divide dough in half and then into five pieces per half, forming each piece into a ball. Roll each ball into a 5½-inch circle, top with ⅓ cup pork filling, bring up sides of dough to enclose, then pinch together and twist. Place on parchment paper. Cover with a damp towel.

7. Place a steamer on top of 8-quart pot of boiling water. Lay a few cabbage leaves on top of the steamer to prevent buns from sticking. Place buns seam side down, about 1-inch apart, on top of leaves. Cover and cook for 15 to 20 minutes or until dough puffs up and is soft and spongy.

8. Serve while hot. These also freeze beautifully.

Clean Meanings

Hoisin sauce is a Chinese sauce usually used as part of a marinade for meats or an ingredient in stir-fries. It is made from fermented or salted soybeans or black beans, sugar, vinegar, garlic, spices, and sweet potato.

Thanksgiving Meatloaf

You can make this turkey meatloaf, which contains all the fixins of a Thanksgiving dinner—sweet potato, dried cranberries, sage, whole wheat bread, celery, and onion—any time of year.

1 package (about 1.3 lb.) lean (at least 93 percent) ground turkey

1 large fresh egg white

1 garlic clove, peeled and crushed

1 small stalk celery, finely chopped

3 fresh sage leaves, finely chopped (about 1 tsp.)

¼ cup dried cranberries

½ medium onion, finely chopped

2 slices of whole wheat bread soaked in ¼ cup water

2 TB. fresh parsley, finely chopped

½ tsp. sea salt

¼ tsp. ground black pepper

3 TB. fine *bulgur*, soaked in ½ cup of hot water for 5 to 10 minutes, then drained

3 sprigs thyme (about ½ tsp.), finely chopped

½ tsp. orange zest

1 small baked sweet potato, peeled and coarsely chopped

Yield: 12 servings
Prep time: 20 minutes
Cook time: 50 to 55 minutes
Serving size: 1 slice
Each serving has:
207 calories
9 g total fat
2 g saturated fat
20 g protein
13 g carbohydrate
5 g sugars
78 mg cholesterol
2 g fiber
340 mg sodium

1. Heat oven to 350°F. Spray a 9×5-inch loaf pan with cooking spray.

2. Place all ingredients except for sweet potato in large bowl. Mix with wooden spoon or your hands until thoroughly blended.

3. Gently fold in sweet potato. Shape into a loaf, and place in pan. Cover with aluminum foil and bake for 20 minutes. Uncover and cook another 30 to 35 minutes, until lightly brown and internal temperature registers 165°F.

4. Remove from oven, slice into 12 pieces, and serve immediately. This goes great with Maple Veggie Mashed Potatoes (see recipe in Chapter 20).

 Clean Meanings

Bulgur is whole wheat that has been steamed or parboiled, then ground into one of four distinct sizes, (fine, medium, coarse, and whole). It is common in Turkish and Middle Eastern cuisine. Because fine bulgur is ground into such small pieces, you don't have to cook it. All you have to do is rehydrate it with water.

Light Garden Lasagna

Everyone loves lasagna, and this clean version is sure to please with layers of cheese, spinach, mushrooms, and a ground turkey meat sauce. It's a winner every time.

Yield: 8 servings	
Prep time: 15 minutes	
Cook time: 1 hour 5 minutes	
Serving size: 1 (3¼ by 4½-inch) piece	

Each serving has:

373 calories

11 g total fat

4 g saturated fat

26 g protein

51 g carbohydrate

8 g sugars

45 mg cholesterol

8 g fiber

395 mg sodium

1 (13¼-oz.) package whole wheat lasagna noodles

½ lb. lean ground chicken

3 cups Basic Tomato Sauce (see recipe earlier in this chapter)

1 cup low-fat cottage cheese

1 cup part-skim ricotta cheese

2 TB. Pecorino Romano or Parmesan cheese, grated

1 TB. fresh oregano leaves, minced

1 TB. fresh basil, minced

1 egg white

½ cup onion, chopped

1 (8-oz.) package white mushrooms or ½ cup white and ½ cup crimini mushrooms

10 oz. baby spinach (about 15 cups loosely packed)

1. Heat oven to 400°F. Bring 6 quarts of water to a rapid boil over high heat in an 8-quart saucepot. Drop in whole wheat lasagna noodles, two or three pieces at a time. Stir. Return to a rapid boil. Cook for 10 minutes. Drain. Lay noodles flat on waxed paper or aluminum foil to keep from sticking together.

2. While lasagna is cooking, heat a 2-quart saucepot over medium-high heat. Spray with cooking spray. Brown ground chicken, stirring occasionally, 5 to 8 minutes. When chicken is cooked, add tomato sauce. Bring to a boil, reduce heat, and simmer 5 minutes, covered.

3. In a large bowl beat cottage cheese, ricotta, Pecorino Romano, oregano, basil, and egg white until smooth. Set aside.

4. Spray small sauté pan with cooking spray and heat over medium-high heat. Add onion and mushrooms, cook for 2 or 3 minutes until soft. Mix in spinach, tossing frequently until wilted. Take off the stove.

5. To assemble, spread ½ cup sauce on the bottom of 9×13-inch roasting pan. Lay cooked lasagna noodles on top to make one even layer. Spread half the cheese mixture over noodles, then half the spinach-mushroom mixture, and ¾ cup sauce. Repeat noodle, cheese, spinach, and sauce layers. Top with noodles, and finish with remaining sauce.

6. Lay a piece of parchment paper over the top of the lasagna, then cover tightly with foil. Bake for 30 minutes. Remove foil and parchment paper and bake another 20 to 25 minutes, until brown and bubbly. Serve hot.

Wholesome Habits

If you're concerned about high blood pressure, be sure to include low-fat dairy products in your diet—about 3 servings a day. These foods are high in calcium and magnesium, two minerals important for controlling blood pressure.

Roast Turkey Breast with Lemon and Oregano

You won't be able to resist the aroma of this roast turkey drenched in lemon and oregano. It's a perfect meal for a big Sunday dinner or when company is coming over. Leftovers make great turkey sandwiches.

Yield: 27 servings

Prep time: 5 minutes

Cook time: 3 hours

Serving size: 3 ounces turkey

Each serving has:

131 calories

3 g total fat

1 g saturated fat

24 g protein

0 g carbohydrate

0 g sugars

75 mg cholesterol

0 g fiber

66 mg sodium

1 whole bone-in turkey breast (legs and thighs removed), 8 to 10 lb.	**Zest of 1 large lemon (about 2 tsp.)**
¼ tsp. sea salt	**2 tsp. extra-virgin olive oil**
¼ tsp. ground black pepper	**1 TB. fresh oregano, finely chopped**
Juice of 1 large lemon (about 4 TB. total)	**2 garlic cloves, peeled and crushed**

1. Heat oven to 350°F. Clean excess fat from turkey and rinse with water. Place in large roasting pan, breast up. Sprinkle with salt, pepper, and 2 tablespoons of lemon juice.

2. Roast in oven uncovered for 1½ hours, basting with pan juices every 30 minutes.

3. In a small bowl mix remaining lemon juice, lemon zest, olive oil, oregano, and garlic. After turkey has cooked for 1½ hours, remove it from oven and brush on all of the lemon-oregano mixture. Cover turkey with aluminum foil. Return to oven for another 1 to 1½ hours, until interior reaches a temperature of 165°F and juices run clear when poked with a fork.

4. Remove breast meat from bone using a sharp knife (save the bones for stock). Place on cutting board, slice into thin slices and serve immediately.

Variation: For a more French-inspired turkey, try replacing the oregano with fresh tarragon leaves.

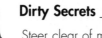 **Dirty Secrets**

Steer clear of meats labeled "enhanced with 15 percent solution" or "contains up to 15 percent natural chicken broth." This is just another way of saying your poultry has been injected with a salt (and sometimes a salt-sugar) solution, which can add as much as 140 milligram of sodium to each 4-ounce breast.

Rosemary Roast Beef

What could be more comforting than a roast beef? Simply dressed with garlic and rosemary, this protein will be the star of the meal. Dress it up with a baked sweet potato or Maple Veggie Mashed Potatoes (see recipe in Chapter 20) and Egg-stra Special Cauliflower (see recipe in Chapter 19) and impress your family and friends.

3 lb. beef eye round roast	**⅛ tsp. ground black pepper**
4 garlic cloves, peeled and cut in half	**¼ tsp. sea salt**
1 tsp. olive oil	**1 cup water**
	1 whole stem rosemary

Yield: 16 servings
Prep time: 5 minutes
Cook time: 2 hours
Serving size: 3 ounce serving
Each serving has:
140 calories
4 g total fat
1 g saturated fat
25 g protein
0 g carbohydrate
0 g sugars
45 mg cholesterol
0 g fiber
69 mg sodium

1. Heat oven to 325°F. Trim any excess fat off eye round. Make 8 (1½-inch deep) cuts in meat with paring knife. Insert half garlic clove into each cut.

2. Rub meat with olive oil, black pepper, and sea salt. Heat a large skillet over medium-high heat. When hot, sear meat on all sides, 1 to 2 minutes on each side.

3. Place meat in a 7×11-inch roasting pan. Deglaze skillet with 1 cup water, scraping up bits with a wooden spoon. Then pour mixture over roast beef in pan. Remove leaves from rosemary stem and coarsely chop. Rub into meat.

4. Place in oven and roast for 1½ to 1¾ hours, or until internal temperature registers 135°F (for a medium doneness). Let meat rest for 15 to 20 minutes, internal temperature will rise to 145°F. Slice thinly and serve.

Wholesome Habits

Beef continues to cook even after it's out of the oven. That's why most meats should be removed from the oven slightly undercooked. Internal temperature can actually rise 10 degrees upon standing for 15 to 20 minutes.

Orange Beef Stew

This powerhouse beef stew is brimming with beta-carotene, thanks to plenty of carrots, sweet potatoes, and acorn squash. Livened up with a splash of orange juice, it is pure comfort food with a clean, nutritious twist.

Yield: 6 cups
Prep time: 15 minutes
Cook time: 1 hour
Serving size: 1½ cup serving
Each serving has:
391 calories
7 g total fat
2 g saturated fat
52 g protein
24 g carbohydrate
4 g sugars
100 mg cholesterol
3 g fiber
359 mg sodium

2 tsp. olive oil

1 lb. beef eye round, cut into 1-inch cubes

⅔ medium onion, diced

2 medium stalks celery, diced

2 medium carrots, cut into 1-inch dice

2 garlic cloves, peeled and minced

8 tsp. whole wheat flour

4 cups Homemade Beef Stock (see recipe in Chapter 17)

1 tsp. fresh sage, chopped

1 tsp. fresh thyme, chopped

¼ tsp. ground black pepper

½ tsp. kosher salt

Juice from 1 orange (4 TB.)

Zest from 1 orange (2 tsp.)

2 large bay leaves

1 small sweet potato, peeled and cut into 1-inch cubes

½ lb. acorn squash, peeled and cut into 1-inch cubes

1. Heat olive oil in a large stock pot over medium-high heat. Brown meat in pan for about 3 minutes and remove.

2. Add onion, celery, carrot, and garlic. Cook, covered, for 2 minutes. Stir in flour and cook for 2 more minutes.

3. Mix in beef stock, sage, thyme, black pepper, salt, orange juice, zest, bay leaves, and cooked beef. Bring to a boil. Reduce heat to low, cover, and simmer for 25 minutes.

4. Add sweet potato and acorn squash. Cover and simmer another 30 minutes or until all vegetables are tender. Remove bay leaves. Serve hot.

Variation: You can make this stew with white potatoes, turnips, rutabagas, parsnips, beets, zucchini, green beans, peas, or any other vegetable. Just make sure to add at least 4 cups of vegetables total.

Wholesome Habits _____

Beta-carotene is a form of vitamin A only found in plants. Among its many benefits, it helps ward off infection by boosting your immune function. Most people know about the orange or yellow vegetables high in beta-carotene, but green vegetables like kale, collards, broccoli, and asparagus are also good sources of this nutrient.

18

Doing Double Duty: Two-in-One Meals

In This Chapter

◆ Cooking once, eating twice

◆ Creating your own convenience foods

◆ Recipes with an international flair

No doubt about it, we live in a fast-paced world, where everyone wants everything done right now. Think of the immediacy of instant messaging, cell phones, and the Internet. When it comes to eating dinner, we want that same instant gratification, which is why processed foods have become so popular. They provide us with food fast.

Clean eaters face the same time challenges as anyone else, and while you may occasionally opt for a frozen meal, for the most part you won't be sacrificing good nutrition (or taste) for convenience. The truth is that you don't have to. As you become more accustomed to cooking clean, you'll develop your own set of kitchen shortcuts, specifically designed with your family in mind, creating a "bank" of your favorite go-to dinners for busy nights.

To get you thinking clean and thinking ahead, we've taken one of the many clean cooking strategies in this book and highlighted it in this chapter. We call it *doing double duty,* and it means cooking two meals (or part of a meal) at one time. The first meal is to be eaten at the time you make it, and the second is reserved for use a few days or weeks (if you freeze it) down the road. For example, Easy Baked Fish Sticks served with Maple Veggie Mashed Potatoes and steamed peas one day morphs into Mexican Fish Tortillas, dressed with a broccoli-cabbage slaw and rolled in a whole wheat tortilla, on another day. Similarly, Pork Tenderloin with Cherry Sauce reappears on the table as Wild Rice Pork Pilaf a few days later. We give you 5 double duty meals (10 recipes altogether) in this chapter.

While these recipes center on the protein portion of the meal, roasted vegetables, starches, and beans can do double duty just as well. Once you get the hang of it, you'll find yourself planning two—and maybe even three or four—meals with one single ingredient. Preplanning these foods will not only save you time and ensure you and your family are getting a healthy, nutritious meal, this strategy can save you money, too. First, because it allows you to buy in bulk, which costs less, and second because you'll waste less food. What could be better than that!

Avocado and Corn Crab Cakes

Avocado, corn, and cilantro keep these oven-baked crab cakes moist and flavorful as well as low in fat and calories. Enjoy with sweet Peach Maple Jam (see recipe in Chapter 11).

1 lb. lump blue crabmeat, picked over for shells	2 green onions (about ¼ cup), chopped
1 whole, fresh egg	½ tsp. fresh mustard or ¼ tsp. dry mustard
2 slices whole wheat bread, processed into breadcrumbs	⅛ tsp. black pepper
6 TB. ground whole wheat crackers (3 whole Matzo crackers or 12 whole wheat crackers)	½ tsp. hot sauce (optional)
	½ cup diced avocado
	½ cup corn, thawed from frozen
⅓ cup nonfat, plain Greek yogurt	1 tsp. lime juice
	2 tsp. finely chopped cilantro

Yield: 8 servings
Prep time: 15 minutes
Cook time: 10 minutes
Serving size: 1 crab cake
Each serving has:
145 calories
4 g total fat
1 g saturated fat
15 g protein
13 g carbohydrate
2 g sugars
83 mg cholesterol
2 g fiber
238 mg sodium

1. Heat oven to 475°F. In a large bowl, gently mix crab with egg, breadcrumbs, 2 tablespoons ground whole wheat crackers, and yogurt. Add green onions, mustard, pepper, hot sauce (if using), avocado, corn, lime juice, and cilantro, and fold together.

2. Measure out ½-cup portions for each crab cake. Form into ½-inch thick patties.

3. Place remaining cracker crumbs in a small bowl. Coat each crab cake well on both sides with crumbs, then place on baking sheet or baking stone sprayed with cooking spray. Lightly spray tops of crab cakes with cooking spray then bake in oven 10 minutes or until golden brown. Serve immediately.

Variation: If you want something sweeter try these substitutions: replace avocado and corn with ½ cup chopped mango and ¼ cup chopped sweet red pepper. Replace the cilantro with 2 teaspoons chopped fresh dill and use 1 teaspoon lime juice instead of lemon juice. Serve on a bed of shredded cucumber.

Clean Cuts _____

Blue crabmeat is available canned fresh (refrigerated) or shelf-stable (pasteurized). Unless you live in a coastal region or have a very good relationship with your fishmonger, I would go for pasteurized product. Read the label to be sure there are no chemicals or bleaches added. Jumbo lump is the most expensive and has the largest-size pieces, but for this recipe, lump (sometimes called backfin) or white meat crab is better and cheaper.

Citrus-Scented Cod Topped with Crab

Make extra crab cakes so you can use them as a topping for this mild white fish dish, which is baked with three zesty citrus juices.

16 oz. cod, cut into 4 fillets

4 (2-oz. scoops) Avocado and Corn Crab Cake mixture, uncooked

1 tsp. extra-virgin olive oil

Juice and zest of 1 orange (about ¼ cup orange juice and 1 TB. orange zest)

Juice and zest of ½ lemon (about 2 TB. juice and 2 tsp. zest)

Juice and zest of ½ lime (about 1 TB. juice and 1 tsp. zest)

1 TB. fresh parsley, chopped

Kosher salt (optional)

Dash ground pepper

Yield: 4 servings
Prep time: 10 minutes
Cook time: 10 minutes
Serving size: 4 ounces cod with 2 ounces crab topping
Each serving has:
266 calories
6 g total fat
1 g saturated fat
35 g protein
18 g carbohydrate
5 g sugars
131 mg cholesterol
2 g fiber
299 mg sodium

1. Heat oven to 375°F. Place cod fillets on a cookie sheet sprayed with cooking spray or stoneware. Top each fillet with 2 ounces of uncooked Avocado and Corn Crab Cake mixture.

2. In a small bowl whisk together olive oil, orange juice and zest, lemon juice and zest, lime juice and zest, and parsley. Pour evenly over fish fillets. Sprinkle with salt (if using) and black pepper. Bake 8 to 10 minutes or until fish flakes easily with a fork and crab cake mixture is cooked through.

3. Serve immediately. You can also freeze cod with crab topping, uncooked; before baking, thaw fish in refrigerator for several hours.

Wholesome Habits

There are more than 50 varieties of avocados, but the best known types in the United States are the Hass avocado, grown in California, and the Mexico or Florida avocado. Hass avocados are soft and buttery with a dark purple, bumpy skin. Florida and Mexico avocados are usually much larger with glossy green skin and about half the fat of Hass. Either one is a good choice. Not only are avocados high in "good" monounsaturated fats, they're also rich in fiber, potassium, folate, and niacin.

Beef Tenderloin with Asparagus and Toasted Barley

Hearty and satisfying is the best way to describe this colorful stir-fry, which features tender strips of beef tossed with tomatoes, onions, and asparagus served over toasted barley for a good dose of fiber.

Yield: 2 servings
Prep time: 15 minutes
Cook time: 25 minutes
Serving size: 1 cup vegetable-meat mixture and 1 cup barley mixture
Each serving has:
337 calories
6 g total fat
2 g saturated fat
20 g protein
54 g carbohydrate
10 g sugars
34 mg cholesterol
8 g fiber
331 mg sodium

⅔ cup quick cooking barley

1⅓ cups plus 2 TB. water

1 tsp. olive oil

4 oz. beef tenderloin or strip steak, cut into ½-inch by 2-inch strips

6 oz. asparagus, cut on a bias in 1½-inch pieces (about 11 medium spears)

¼ medium onion, sliced

1 garlic clove, peeled and minced

½ cup tart cherry juice or balsamic vinegar

½ medium tomato, diced

1 tsp. thyme leaves or any herb you like, finely chopped

⅛ tsp. ground black pepper

¼ tsp. sea salt

1. Toast barley in a large skillet over medium heat for 5 to 7 minutes or until it releases a nutty aroma and begins turning brown.

2. Put 1⅓ cups water in a 2-quart saucepot and bring to a boil. Mix in barley. Cover and return to boiling; reduce heat to a simmer and cook 12 minutes. Remove from heat and let stand 5 minutes.

3. Rinse the skillet you toasted the barley in and use to heat olive oil over medium-high heat. Add beef and brown for about 3 minutes. Stir frequently. Remove meat to a plate, cover, and set aside.

4. In same skillet sauté asparagus, onion, garlic, and cherry juice. Cook, covered, about 2 minutes over medium-high heat. Asparagus will begin to soften. Return beef to the pan, along with tomato, thyme, pepper, and salt. Cook for another minute or two, adding a tablespoon or two of water, if necessary.

5. To serve, place 1 cup barley in each of two bowls. Pour about 1 cup vegetable beef mixture over top. Serve immediately.

Wholesome Habits

Like most whole grains, barley is high in B vitamins, including niacin, and copper, but where it really shines is its fiber content. Cup for cup, barley has twice as much fiber as brown rice and six times more than white rice.

Warm Tuscan Beef Salad

Using left over beef tenderloin and precooked roasted beets is the key to getting this hearty, rustic salad on the table in minutes. It's finished with a basil-garlic dressing laced with tart cherry juice and a sprinkle of blue cheese.

4 cups arugula or spinach or any dark mild green

4 cups Butterhead or Bibb lettuce, chopped

8 oz. fennel bulb, thinly sliced (about 2 cups)

2 cups blanched green beans, cut into 1½-inch pieces

4 small beets, roasted, peeled, and diced

½ lb. cooked beef tenderloin, cubed

1 oz. (about 1 TB.) blue cheese crumbled (optional)

¼ tsp. ground black pepper

Dressing:

12 basil leaves (about 4 TB. chopped)

1 garlic clove, peeled

2 TB. red onion, chopped

2 tsp. lemon juice

2 tsp. balsamic vinegar

4 TB. tart or sweet cherry juice

2 TB. extra-virgin olive oil

Yield: 4 servings
Prep time: 10 minutes
Cook time: 5 minutes
Serving size: 2 cups of salad, 2 tablespoons dressing
Each serving has:
251 calories
12 g total fat
3 g saturated fat
20 g protein
18 g carbohydrate
9 g sugars
41 mg cholesterol
5 g fiber
127 mg sodium

1. In four large serving bowls, layer arugula, lettuce, fennel, green beans, and beets. Heat beef in a small sauté pan over medium heat until warm. Place ¼ of the beef on each salad. Sprinkle with blue cheese (if using) and pepper.

2. Put all dressing ingredients in a small food processor. Process on high for 20 seconds until blended. Pour 2 tablespoons of dressing on each salad. Serve.

Variation: You can replace the plain beets in this recipe with 2 cups of leftover Sweet Beets with Walnuts and Chèvre (see recipe in Chapter 19).

Clean Cuts

There couldn't be anything easier than roasting beets. Just wash them well (you don't have to peel them), cut off the ends, wrap them in foil, and bake in a 375°F oven for 1 to 1½ hours (depending on size) until tender when poked with fork. Let cool, slip off skin, and dice.

Easy Baked Fish Sticks

Cornmeal mixed with whole wheat breadcrumbs gives these low-fat fish sticks their crunch, while chili powder spices them up.

Yield: 4 servings
Prep time: 15 minutes
Cook time: 12 minutes
Serving size: 6 to 8 fish sticks (4 ounces total)
Each serving has:
194 calories
4 g total fat
1 g saturated fat
27 g protein
13 g carbohydrate
1 g sugars
56 mg cholesterol
2 g fiber
158 mg sodium

Wholesome Habits

Tilapia is a lean white fish with a firm flesh and mild taste. It's native to the Middle East and Africa, and in the United States only farm-raised tilapia is available. You'll find it in the fish section at most grocery stores.

1 lb. tilapia or other firm white fish	1 tsp. fresh parsley chopped or ½ tsp. dried
2 slices whole wheat bread, crust removed	½ tsp. paprika
¼ cup stone-ground yellow cornmeal	½ tsp. chili powder
	¼ tsp. sea salt (optional)
1 tsp. garlic powder	1 tsp. olive oil
1 tsp. onion powder	2 fresh large egg whites
¼ tsp. ground black pepper	1 TB. water

1. Heat oven to 425°F. Spray a cookie sheet with cooking spray or use baking stoneware (stone does not need to be sprayed). Cut tilapia into 1-inch strips (about ½-ounce pieces) and set aside on a plate.

2. Place bread in a food processor and process on high about 10 to 15 seconds until fine crumbs form. Add cornmeal, garlic powder, onion powder, pepper, parsley, paprika, chili powder, salt (if using), and olive oil. Pulse 5 or 6 times (about 15 seconds) until thoroughly mixed. Mixture should be crumbly.

3. Pour breadcrumb mixture into a shallow bowl. In another shallow bowl beat together egg whites and water.

4. On a flat work surface, line up the fish, egg mixture, breadcrumb mixture, and cookie sheet. In several batches, place a few strips of fish in egg white mixture and coat, roll fish in breadcrumb mixture until all surfaces are covered, then place fish on the cookie sheet.

5. Bake for 12 minutes, or until fish flakes with fork. Serve with clean ketchup (see recipe in Chapter 21), potatoes, sweet potato fries, or brown rice and a vegetable. Make extra and save for Mexican Fish Tortillas (see the following recipe).

Mexican Fish Tortillas

Inspired by the fish taco joints popular in Southern California, crunchy fish sticks are wrapped in a whole wheat tortilla with shredded cabbage and broccoli slaw. Jalapeños and salsa give this dish its kick.

8 cooked Easy Baked Fish Sticks (see recipe earlier in this chapter)

1 cup packaged broccoli slaw

1 cup white cabbage, shredded

½ tsp. jalapeño pepper, finely chopped (optional)

2 TB. low-sodium organic salsa

2 TB. low-fat sour cream

1 tsp. fresh cilantro, chopped

1 tsp. lime juice

2 whole wheat flour tortillas

Yield: 2 servings
Prep time: 10 minutes
Cook time: 10 minutes
Serving size: 1 fish tortilla
Each serving has:
278 calories
6 g total fat
1 g saturated fat
20 g protein
39 g carbohydrate
6 g sugars
33 mg cholesterol
7 g fiber
522 mg sodium

1. Heat oven to 400°F. Wrap fish sticks in aluminum foil and bake for 10 to 15 minutes or until warm. You can also microwave the fish sticks for 1 to 2 minutes or until heated through.

2. In a small bowl, mix together broccoli slaw, cabbage, jalapeño (if using), salsa, sour cream, cilantro, and lime juice.

3. Warm tortillas in the microwave on high for 10 to 15 seconds.

4. On a flat work surface place one flour tortilla. In center of tortilla place 1 cup slaw mixture, leaving 1-inch around the edge of the tortilla. Top with one fish stick. Fold bottom of tortilla over fish and slaw, then tuck in each side and roll up.

Clean Cuts

You can make up a big batch of these fish sticks a day or two in advance, for two meals in one week, or you can precook and freeze them. Then all you have to do is pull them out of the fridge or freezer and reheat them for the Mexican Fish Tortillas.

Honey Spiced Chicken

Fragrant Indian spices, sweet honey, and black tea flavor this chicken, which will attract as many fans for its wonderful aroma as it will for its taste. Prepare it a few hours in advance, or even the night before, so the chicken has time to absorb the flavors.

Yield: 4 servings
Prep time: 5 minutes, plus at least 1 hour for marinating
Cook time: 15 minutes
Serving size: 4 ounces chicken

Each serving has:
185 calories
3 g total fat
1 g saturated fat
34 g protein
4 g carbohydrate
4 g sugars
87 mg cholesterol
0 g fiber
97 mg sodium

1 lb. boneless, skinless chicken breast, cut into 4 cutlets

1 tsp. *garam masala*

2 tsp. honey

1 TB. prepared black tea

½ tsp. extra-virgin olive oil

1. Place chicken cutlets in small bowl along with garam masala, honey, tea, and olive oil. Mix well, then put in refrigerator and let marinate for at least one hour or overnight.

2. Heat oven to high broil. Place marinated chicken on dry stoneware or cookie sheet sprayed with cooking oil. Broil for 10 to 15 minutes, until done, depending on how thick your chicken pieces are. Serve with your favorite vegetable or starch. This chicken goes well with nearly everything.

 Clean Meanings _____

> **Garam masala** is a popular Indian spice blend available at many mainstream grocery stores and natural food stores. Recipes vary widely, but if you want to make it yourself, here's a quick fix: in a small bowl combine 1 teaspoon each of ground cardamom, cumin, coriander, and black pepper with ½ teaspoon cinnamon and ¼ teaspoon ground cloves. Blend well, seal tightly in a glass jar, and store with the rest of your spices.

BBQ Chicken Pizza

This dish combines two of America's favorite foods—pizza and barbecue—and is the epitome of the American melting pot. Here our whole wheat clean pizza crust is topped with homemade barbecue sauce, mozzarella cheese, and cooked honey spiced chicken.

1 recipe Whole Wheat Pizza Dough (see recipe in Chapter 17)

½ cup Homemade BBQ Sauce (see recipe in Chapter 21)

½ lb. cooked Honey Spiced Chicken (see recipe earlier in this chapter)

4 ounces part-skim mozzarella, grated (about 1 cup)

Yield: 6 servings (12 slices)
Prep time: 5 minutes
Cook time: 12 to 15 minutes
Serving size: 2 slices each
Each serving has:
445 calories
13 g total fat
3 g saturated fat
24 g protein
62 g carbohydrate
7 g sugars
34 mg cholesterol
10 g fiber
278 mg sodium

1. Heat oven to 425°F. Roll out pizza dough to fit a large baking stone (15×10½-inches) or cookie sheet. Spread BBQ sauce over top, then top with Honey Spiced Chicken and cheese.

2. Bake for 12 to 15 minutes or until cheese starts to brown.

3. Serve hot right out of the oven.

Variation: You can also make this pizza with store-bought whole wheat pizza dough. Use two packages of dough in place of 1 recipe of Whole Wheat Pizza Dough. Because sodium levels are higher, serving size is 1 slice.

Dirty Secrets

Fast food pizza is about as "unclean" as you can get. Just two slices are loaded with fat, saturated fat, and more than a day's worth of sodium, not to mention a hefty supply of calories—and that's just cheese pizza! Pepperoni, sausage, olives, and other toppings make the numbers soar even higher.

Pork Tenderloin with Cherry Sauce

Pork tenderloin is an extremely lean and tender cut of meat. A light dried cherry sauce adds a splash of color and sweetness.

Yield: 6 servings
Prep time: 10 minutes
Cook time: 35 minutes
Serving size: 4 ounces pork with 2 tablespoons cherry sauce
Each serving has:
212 calories
6 g total fat
2 g saturated fat
30 g protein
8 g carbohydrate
6 g sugars
82 mg cholesterol
0 g fiber
161 mg sodium

1½ lb. pork tenderloin	1 TB. all-natural fruit-sweetened black cherry fruit spread
¼ tsp. sea salt	
⅛ tsp. ground black pepper	1 tsp. balsamic vinegar
⅛ tsp. garlic powder	¼ cup dried tart (unsweetened) red cherries, coarsely chopped
2 tsp. extra-virgin olive oil	
2 TB. onion, finely chopped	
½ cup water	⅛ tsp. ground black pepper

1. Heat oven to 450°F. Spray a 9×12-inch roasting pan with cooking spray. Remove any excess fat from pork. Season with salt, black pepper, and garlic powder and rub with 1 teaspoon olive oil. Place pork in the roasting pan, uncovered, and cook for 30 minutes or until juices run clear when poked with a fork and internal temperature reaches 150°F.

2. Remove cooked pork from oven and place on a serving plate to rest for 10 minutes (internal temperature should rise to 160°F). Set roasting pan aside.

3. To make sauce, sauté onion and remaining olive oil in small saucepan. Place roasting pan on burner and heat over medium-high heat and *deglaze* pan with water, fruit spread, and balsamic vinegar, stirring to scrape up bits of browned pork from the bottom of the pan. Bring to a boil, stirring constantly, for 1 to 2 minutes. Pour into saucepan with onion and add dried cherries and pepper. Bring to boil for about 30 seconds, and remove from heat.

4. Cut pork tenderloin into thin (1-ounce) slices and serve 4 slices with 2 tablespoons dried cherry sauce. This dish is excellent with roasted or mashed potatoes, brussels sprouts, or green beans.

Clean Meanings

Deglaze is a term chefs use to describe the process of scraping up and mixing with a liquid the bits of browned meat left in the pan after meat has been sautéed, roasted, or broiled. Deglazed sauces are simple and flavorful. They can also be lighter and lower in calories than traditional sauces.

Wild Rice Pork Pilaf

Using leftover pork tenderloin and precooked rice is the key to having this meal on the table in minutes. To complete the meal, the rice and pork are tossed with colorful vegetables and a flavorful spice mix.

2 tsp. olive oil

¼ cup onion, diced

1 cup sliced mushrooms

3 cups shredded spinach

8 oz. (about 1 cup) cooked Pork Tenderloin (see recipe earlier in this chapter), diced

4 cups cooked Wild Rice Blend (see recipe in Chapter 20)

½ cup diced tomato

1 TB. fresh basil, chopped

1 TB. Eating Clean Spice Blend (see recipe in Chapter 21)

⅛ tsp. sea salt (optional)

Hot sauce (optional)

Yield: 4 servings
Prep time: 15 minutes
Cook time: 10 minutes
Serving size: 1½ cups
Each serving has:
305 calories
6 g total fat
1 g saturated fat
21 g protein
41 g carbohydrate
2 g sugars
41 mg cholesterol
4 g fiber
105 mg sodium

1. Heat olive oil in a large sauté pan over medium-high heat. Add onion, mushrooms, and spinach, and cook for 2 to 3 minutes until vegetables begin to get soft.

2. Add pork and cook 1 minute. Gently mix in wild rice, tomato, basil, spice blend, and salt (if using). Cook for 5 to 10 more minutes until heated through.

3. Serve with hot sauce (if using).

Wholesome Habits

Though commonly used to refer to rice, a pilaf is any whole grain cooked with a variety of vegetables and meats. The dish, which originated in the Middle East, dates back to the fifth century and inspired the likes of paella, jambalaya, fried rice, and risotto.

Chapter 19

Star Vegetable Sides

In This Chapter

- ◆ Oven-roasting vegetables
- ◆ Steaming side dishes
- ◆ Dressy veggies for any occasion

Everyone knows vegetables are an essential part of healthful eating, but for clean eaters these colorful side dishes deserve special attention, mainly because they demand it. Yes, cooking with fresh-from-the-farmers'-market vegetables requires a bit more planning and prep time than using canned, frozen, or convenience produce, but in return you'll be rewarded with fresher, brighter, more intense flavors.

In most of these recipes you'll notice that salt, if included at all, is usually optional. That's because as you become more accustomed to eating clean you'll begin to appreciate the natural sweetness of the vegetable. You may even discover that you don't need to add any salt!

To give you an idea of what the world of produce has to offer, we've included a variety of vegetables—from winter beets to summer zucchini—prepared in a number of ways ranging from the set-it-and-forget-it type recipes like Baked Butternut Squash to the more complex dishes like Crunchy Carrot Soufflé.

Our focus is on clean cooking methods, like blanching, baking, steaming, roasting, and sautéing, which bring out flavor without compromising taste or nutrition. We also show you techniques for seasoning your vegetables with natural clean aromatics like fresh herbs, citrus zest, and nuts.

Even if you are not a big vegetable fan, it pays to become more adventuresome with produce. Try something new, explore unusual combinations, or simply put a new twist on family favorites. Most of all, taste it. You just may like it.

Oven Roasted Brussels Sprouts

Baking brussels sprouts on high heat turns them brown and crispy on the outside and moist and tender on the inside. They're so good you'll want to eat them like candy.

1 lb. brussels sprouts, cleaned and washed, bottom trimmed and halved

1 TB. olive oil

1 TB. honey

¼ tsp. salt (optional)

⅛ tsp. crushed red pepper

Yield: 4 cups
Prep time: 10 minutes
Cook time: 25 minutes
Serving size: 1 cup
Each serving has:
97 calories
1 g total fat
0 g saturated fat
4 g protein
15 g carbohydrate
7 g sugars
0 mg cholesterol
4 g fiber
174 mg sodium

1. Heat oven to 450°F. Spray a 9×13-inch roasting pan with cooking spray.

2. Toss brussels sprouts with olive oil and honey in the prepared roasting pan. Sprinkle with salt (if using) and red pepper.

3. Cook for 25 minutes or until leaves turn brown and crispy.

Variation: Vary the sweetener or skip it altogether and instead drizzle the brussels sprouts with 1 tablespoon balsamic vinegar. Or omit the olive oil, spray with cooking spray instead, and add 1 tablespoon finely chopped nuts. These brussels sprouts can also be substituted for the beets in the Warm Tuscan Beef Salad (see recipe in Chapter 18).

Wholesome Habits

One cup of brussels sprouts has more vitamin C than an orange, providing more than 100 percent of your recommended daily allowance. They are also a good source of vitamin K, folate, and potassium.

Baked Butternut Squash

Butternut squash has a smooth, velvety texture and rich, buttery taste. Most people sprinkle it with brown sugar, but we've nixed the sweets in favor of fragrant rosemary and garlic.

Yield: 4 servings
Prep time: 10 minutes
Cook time: 40 minutes
Serving size: 1 cup
Each serving has:
137 calories
3 g total fat
0 g saturated fat
3 g protein
30 g carbohydrate
6 g sugars
0 mg cholesterol
5 g fiber
11 mg sodium

2 lb. butternut squash, peeled, seeded, and cut into 1-inch cubes

4 large garlic cloves, peeled and sliced

½ medium onion, finely chopped

2 tsp. fresh rosemary, finely chopped

2 tsp. extra-virgin olive oil

¼ tsp. ground black pepper

⅛ tsp. sea salt (optional)

1. Heat oven to 375°F. Spray a large roasting pan with cooking spray. Place butternut squash, garlic, onion, and rosemary in the pan and mix. Drizzle with olive oil and sprinkle with black pepper and salt (if using). Gently toss the mixture.

2. Cover tightly with aluminum foil. Bake in oven for 40 minutes.

3. Remove from oven and uncover. Place in serving dish. Serve with chicken, fish, or pork.

Variation: This recipe is used in the Crab and Butternut Squash Bisque (see recipe in Chapter 15). You could also use it in place of acorn squash in Wild Rice and Acorn Squash Pilaf (see recipe in Chapter 23) and in Orange Beef Stew (see recipe in Chapter 17) or it could replace the baked sweet potato in the Thanksgiving Meatloaf (see recipe in Chapter 17).

Wholesome Habits

Butternut squash is only one of the many varieties of squash referred to as winter squash. It is available late summer, autumn, and winter. You can substitute any kind of summer or winter squash in this recipe.

Sesame Broccoli

In this Asian-inspired dish, lightly steamed broccoli is drizzled with sesame oil then tossed with sesame seeds, grated ginger, and crushed red pepper.

1 cup water	1 tsp. sesame seeds
1 lb. broccoli, cut into small pieces	1 tsp. fresh ginger, grated
½ tsp. sesame seed oil	½ tsp. crushed red pepper

Yield: 4 servings
Prep time: 5 minutes
Cook time: 10 minutes
Serving size: 1 cup
Each serving has:
51 calories
2 g total fat
0 g saturated fat
3 g protein
8 g carbohydrate
2 g sugars
0 mg cholesterol
3 g fiber
37 mg sodium

1. Bring water to boil in 4-quart saucepan over medium-high heat. Place broccoli in metal steamer over top of water. Make sure broccoli is about ½- to 1-inch above the boiling water. Cover tightly and cook for 5 to 7 minutes until tender.

2. Place broccoli in a bowl, drizzle with sesame seed oil, then sprinkle with sesame seeds, ginger, and crushed red pepper. Gently toss. Serve hot.

Clean Cuts

Steaming is a gentle, moist cooking method that preserves nutrients as well as texture and flavor. For best results use metal or bamboo steamer, a small amount of water (don't let the liquid touch the food), a tight-fitting lid, and be sure to check water frequently (every 15 minutes) as it can evaporate. Adding garlic, ginger, or fresh herbs to the water imparts a subtle flavor to food.

Garlicky Spinach with Kalamata Olives

Who would have thought that combining two Mediterranean ingredients—roasted garlic and salty kalamata olives—with mild spinach would produce such a delicious side dish. You have to try it to believe it.

Yield: 6 servings
Prep time: 10 minutes
Cook time: 15 minutes
Serving size: ¾ cup
Each serving has:
26 calories
2 g total fat
0 g saturated fat
1 g protein
2 g carbohydrate
0 g sugars
2 mg cholesterol
1 g fiber
72 mg sodium

Olive oil

3 whole garlic cloves, peeled

9 kalamata olives, pitted and chopped

1 (9-oz.) bag or bunch spinach, washed and cleaned

3 TB. water

Cracked black pepper

1. Heat oven to 450°F. Dip your fingers in olive oil and rub on 3 whole garlic cloves. Wrap garlic in aluminum foil and bake in oven for 10 to 12 minutes.

2. Remove garlic from oven. Let cool for a minute or two, then finely chop (garlic will be more like a paste) and toss with kalamata olives. Set aside.

3. Heat a medium-size sauté pan over medium-high heat. Place spinach and 2 tablespoons water in hot pan. Toss continuously with a pair of tongs for about 15 seconds until spinach begins to wilt. Add kalamata olives, garlic, and remaining tablespoon of water if needed, and continue to toss until spinach is cooked through, about 2 minutes total. Sprinkle with cracked black pepper and serve.

Wholesome Habits

Kalamata olives, also called Greek olives, are named after the Kalamata region in Greece. They are dark purple in color and available pitted or unpitted. They're typically high in fat (think olive oil) and sodium, so use small amounts at a time.

Sweet Beets with Walnuts and Chèvre

Roasting beets turns them sweet and tender. Topped with a sprinkle of crunchy walnuts and a crumble of goat cheese, they go from ordinary to elegant.

2 lb. beets, peeled, cut into ½-inch cubes

½ medium onion, chopped (about ½ cup)

3 garlic cloves, peeled and minced

¼ tsp. sea salt (optional)

1 tsp. extra-virgin olive oil

2 TB. chopped toasted walnuts

2 oz. chèvre (soft plain goat cheese), crumbled

Yield: 10 servings
Prep time: 20 minutes
Cook time: 1 hour and 15 minutes
Serving size: ½ cup
Each serving has:
81 calories
4 g total fat
1 g saturated fat
3 g protein
10 g carbohydrate
7 g sugars
3 mg cholesterol
3 g fiber
91 mg sodium

1. Heat oven to 400°F. Spray a 14×10-inch roasting pan with cooking spray. Place beets, onions, garlic, and salt (if using) in roasting pan and toss together gently. Spread the mixture in an even layer and spray with cooking spray.

2. Cover tightly with aluminum foil and bake in oven for about 1 hour or until beets are soft when poked with fork.

3. Uncover beets. Raise oven temperature to 450°F and drizzle with olive oil. Cook for 15 more minutes, until beets begin to get crisp, but not brown.

4. Remove from oven and sprinkle with toasted walnuts and goat cheese. Serve immediately.

Dirty Secrets

Don't be alarmed if your urine turns pink or red after eating beets. This harmless condition, called beeturia, is a result of a pigment called betacyanin (what gives beets their dark purple-red color), passing through your system. Your urine should return to its normal color in a day or two.

Green Beans with Caramelized Onions

Browning onions over medium heat enhances their sweetness and produces a soft, velvety texture—a perfect match for crisp, crunchy green beans.

Yield: 2 servings
Prep time: 10 minutes
Cook time: 15 minutes
Serving size: ¾ cup
Each serving has:
71 calories
2 g total fat
0 g saturated fat
3 g protein
12 g carbohydrate
3 g sugars
0 mg cholesterol
5 g fiber
8 mg sodium

½ lb. fresh green beans, cleaned and stems removed

1 tsp. extra-virgin olive oil

½ medium onion, sliced

Dash of black pepper

Dash of sea salt (optional)

Dash of nutmeg

1. Fill a 4-quart saucepan with 2 quarts of water and heat over medium-high heat until boiling. Drop green beans in boiling water, reduce heat to medium, and simmer for 8 minutes or until cooked but still firm to the touch. Remove beans from pot, place in a bowl, and set aside.

2. In a small sauté pan, heat olive oil over medium-low heat. Place onions in the pan and cover. Cook for 5 to 7 minutes until soft and lightly brown. Add green beans, black pepper, salt (if using), nutmeg, and 2 tablespoons water. Toss together. Cook for 3 more minutes over medium-high heat.

3. Serve immediately.

Wholesome Habits _____

When the natural sugars in onions are slowly heated they turn a rich dark brown color. This process, called caramelization, produces a sweet, nutty flavor.

Lemony Green Tea Asparagus

In this creative recipe, asparagus is first poached in green tea, then sprinkled with lemony whole wheat breadcrumbs and finished under the broiler.

2 cups green tea

1 lb. asparagus, cleaned and trimmed

1 slice whole wheat bread, crust removed

1 tsp. lemon zest

1 tsp. olive oil

1 tsp. Parmesan cheese

Cracked black pepper

Yield: 4 servings
Prep time: 10 minutes
Cook time: 20 minutes
Serving size: 5 to 7 spears per person
Each serving has:
52 calories
2 g total fat
0 g saturated fat
5 g protein
7 g carbohydrate
3 g sugars
0 mg cholesterol
3 g fiber
42 mg sodium

1. Heat green tea and asparagus in a large shallow saucepan over medium heat until liquid reaches a low simmer. Simmer for 6 to 7 minutes until tender when poked with fork. Remove pan from heat and reserve about ¼ cup liquid.

2. Meanwhile heat oven to high broil. Place bread in a small food processor or chopper and process on high until fine crumbs form. Put breadcrumbs in a small bowl and mix together with lemon zest, olive oil, Parmesan cheese, and black pepper.

3. Put asparagus in an oven safe casserole dish. Sprinkle with breadcrumb mixture, then pour ¼ cup liquid over top. Broil on high until breadcrumbs brown, about 30 seconds to a minute. Serve hot.

Clean Cuts

Asparagus season runs from March through June, but the best time to buy fresh asparagus is April. The size depends on variety, not tenderness. White asparagus is sunlight-deprived and has a milder, more delicate taste. To keep asparagus fresh, trim the bottoms and wrap a moist paper towel around the stem ends, then store in the refrigerator. Another option is to stand the stalks upright in two inches of cold water.

Crunchy Carrot Soufflé

Make this carrot *soufflé* when you want to serve something special. Carrots are whipped until they're light and fluffy, sprinkled with sweet spices, then finished off with a crunchy oatmeal nut topping.

Yield: 7 servings
Prep time: 15 minutes
Cook time: 45 minutes
Serving size: ½ cup
Each serving has:
179 calories
9 g total fat
1 g saturated fat
4 g protein
22 g carbohydrate
11 g sugars
30 mg cholesterol
3 g fiber
139 mg sodium

1 lb. carrots (4–5 medium carrots), peeled and cut into 1-inch pieces

½ cup carrot juice

½ cup water

2 TB. maple syrup

1 whole large egg

2 egg whites

1 TB. Sucanat

3 TB. whole wheat flour

1¼ tsp. baking powder

3 TB. plus 1 tsp. olive oil

1 TB. all-natural, unsweetened apple butter

1 tsp. vanilla extract

¼ tsp. cinnamon

⅛ tsp. nutmeg

¼ cup quick cooking dry oatmeal

2 TB. pecans

1. Heat oven to 350°F and spray a 2-quart glass or ceramic casserole dish with cooking spray.

2. In a large saucepot, combine carrots, carrot juice, water, and maple syrup. Bring to a boil, then reduce to medium heat and simmer for about 20 minutes, until carrots are soft.

3. Transfer carrots and juice from cooking pot to a blender or food processor and purée on high until smooth (about 5 minutes), stopping occasionally to scrape down sides. It's best to do this in small batches.

4. Beat egg and egg whites in a separate bowl. Pour into blender with carrots and purée until completely incorporated. Add Sucanat, whole wheat flour, baking powder, 3 tablespoons of olive oil, apple butter, vanilla, cinnamon, and half of nutmeg. Process on high until completely blended and smooth.

5. Pour carrot mixture into the casserole dish. In a small chopper, place oatmeal, pecans, 1 teaspoon olive oil, and a dash of cinnamon and nutmeg. Pulse 7 or 8 times until well blended and coarse crumbs form.

6. Sprinkle oatmeal mixture over carrots. Carefully place in oven. Cook for 30 to 45 minutes until top puffs up. (Don't open the oven door during cooking or soufflé will sink.) Remove from oven when done. You'll know it's done when it is puffed up in the center. Carrot soufflé will naturally begin to drop slightly as it cools.

Clean Meanings

Soufflé is a French word that literally means "puffed up." In the culinary world soufflés can be sweet or savory. A base of vegetables, cheese, or fruit is typically combined with whipped egg whites, which allow the dish to rise in the oven.

Clean Cauliflower Polonaise

In French, *polonaise* means Polish style. Among chefs, it refers to a vegetable dish topped with hardboiled eggs, breadcrumbs, and browned butter. Here is our clean rendition of cauliflower polonaise.

Yield: 4 servings
Prep time: 10 minutes
Cook time: 10 minutes
Serving size: 1 cup
Each serving has:
88 calories
5 g total fat
1 g saturated fat
5 g protein
8 g carbohydrate
3 g sugars
54 mg cholesterol
3 g fiber
79 mg sodium

5 cups water

1 lb. cauliflower (about ½ medium head), cut in 2-inch florets

1 slice whole wheat bread, coarsely chopped

1 TB. fresh parsley, coarsely chopped

1 TB. fresh chives, coarsely chopped

1 garlic clove, peeled and coarsely chopped

2 tsp. grated Parmesan or Grana Padano

2 tsp. extra-virgin olive oil

1 hardboiled egg, peeled and diced

1. In a large pot over medium-high heat, bring water to a boil. Add cauliflower and simmer at a low boil for 5 to 8 minutes until a fork easily pierces the vegetable. (Do not let the cauliflower get mushy.) Drain and set cauliflower aside.

2. In a food processor bowl place bread, parsley, chives, garlic, and cheese. Pulse at high speed about 5 or 6 times until you see small uniform crumbs.

3. Heat olive oil in a large saucepan over medium-high heat. Add cauliflower, egg, and breadcrumbs to pan, stirring constantly until cauliflower is coated. Serve hot.

Wholesome Habits

Although cauliflower is typically snow-white in color, it is chock full of disease-fighting phytochemicals usually associated with more colorful vegetables. It's also an excellent source of vitamin C and fiber. Purple and green varieties (a cross between broccoli and white cauliflower) are also available.

Oven Fried Zucchini Sticks

Who needs fries when you can have zucchini sticks? These crispy treats get their crunch from a combination of whole wheat flour, wheat germ, and cornmeal, while Parmesan cheese and parsley punch up taste.

2 tsp. water

2 egg whites

4 TB. whole wheat flour

2 TB. wheat germ

2 TB. cornmeal

¼ tsp. ground black pepper

4 tsp. Parmesan cheese

2 tsp. chopped fresh parsley

½ tsp. paprika

2 tsp. extra-virgin olive oil

2 medium zucchini (about 1 lb.), cut into ½-inch by 3½-inch strips

Yield: 4 servings
Prep time: 10 minutes
Cook time: 20 minutes
Serving size: about 4 ounces each (about 4–6 pieces)
Each serving has:
114 calories
4 g total fat
1 g saturated fat
6 g protein
16 g carbohydrate
2 g sugars
1 mg cholesterol
3 g fiber
68 mg sodium

1. Heat oven to 425°F. Mix water and egg whites together in a small bowl. Set aside. In a separate bowl, blend flour, wheat germ, cornmeal, black pepper, Parmesan cheese, parsley, paprika, and olive oil.

2. On a clean work surface create a coating line by placing zucchini, egg mixture, and flour/cornmeal mixture in a row. Coat zucchini first in egg mixture, then in flour-cornmeal mixture, and place coated vegetables on a cookie sheet or baking stone sprayed with cooking spray. Bake for 10 minutes, toss vegetables, and bake for another 10 minutes or until fries are lightly brown.

3. Serve immediately with Clean Ketchup or Rojo Pimiento (see recipes in Chapter 21).

Dirty Secrets

Compared to our recipe, typical fried restaurant-style zucchini contains nearly 5 times more fat, 3 times the calories, and more than 10 times the sodium. Which would you choose?

Chapter 20

Stick-to-Your-Ribs Starches

In This Chapter

◆ Multipurpose multigrains

◆ Savory sides you can eat like a meal

◆ Potatoes that pack a punch

Now that you know about the benefits of eating unprocessed whole grains, it's time to put these principles into practice in the kitchen. If you've been eating clean for a while, you're probably already familiar with brown rice, whole grain bread, and whole wheat pasta. The recipes in this chapter will bring you to the next level.

To tempt more timid taste buds we suggest varying the type of rice. Whole grain brown rice is available in short, medium, and long grain varieties. Now it's even possible to find whole grain jasmine, basmati, sushi, and arborio rice. Our Pineapple Brown Rice is the perfect recipe for experimenting with these different types of rice.

If you're ready to explore more exotic grains, cook up a batch of our All-Purpose Multigrain Blend. This mixture is as versatile as white rice, except with more fiber, more vitamins and minerals, and more taste—and just as easy to make. The best part is you can make one big batch and then eat it throughout the week. It freezes well, too.

Some people can't imagine life without mashed potatoes, and the good news is that you don't have to. Without the heavy cream and butter, clean mashed potatoes serve up light and fluffy with true 'tater taste you and your family will love. Pair your potatoes with other vegetables such as the turnips and cauliflower in our Maple Veggie Mashed Potatoes recipe—you'll be able to sneak in even more nutrition.

Sweet potatoes are another winner and are definitely worth serving more than just once or twice a year. High in fiber, vitamin A, and loads of antioxidants, they are a clean eating staple. Just wait till you try the Spicy Sweet Potato Fries and you'll see what we mean!

All-Purpose Multigrain Blend

Tired of potatoes? Keep this all-purpose nutty tasting rice blend on hand and you'll always have a filling and flavorful side to complement any protein. We love it plain but you can dress it up in a million ways.

3¾ cups water	½ cup millet
1 cup long grain brown rice	½ tsp. cracked black pepper
¼ cup soft wheat berries	¼ tsp. sea salt

Yield: 6 cups
Prep time: 5 minutes
Cook time: 50 minutes
Serving size: ½ cup
Each serving has:
101 calories
1 g total fat
0 g saturated fat
3 g protein
21 g carbohydrate
0 g sugars
0 mg cholesterol
2 g fiber
50 mg sodium

1. In a 3-quart saucepot bring 2¾ cups water to boil over high heat. Add brown rice and wheat berries. Reduce heat to simmer, stir, and cover. Cook about 45 to 50 minutes or until both wheat berries and rice are tender to the bite.

2. While rice is cooking, pour dry millet in a small saucepot and heat over medium-high heat for 4 to 6 minutes or until it becomes toasty brown and smells like popcorn (watch out—it may begin to pop), stirring constantly. Meanwhile bring 1 cup water to a boil in another small pot. When millet has browned, slowly pour the toasted grains into the boiling water, being careful to avoid splattering. Reduce heat to simmer, cover, and cook for 15 to 18 minutes.

3. In a large bowl place cooked millet, cooked brown rice, wheat berries, and pepper and salt. Gently mix. Serve immediately. Store any leftovers in an airtight container in the refrigerator or freezer.

Variation: You can add practically any cooked vegetable or meat like chicken, pork, or shrimp, or even dried fruit and nuts to this all-purpose grain mixture and it will be divine. Here are a few of our favorites.

Apples and Onions: In medium-size saucepan, sauté 1 small apple, peeled, seeded, and chopped, with ¼ cup chopped onion, 2 teaspoons honey, and ⅓ cup low-sodium chicken broth for 5 to 10 minutes until onions and apples are soft. Add 2 cups grain mixture. Heat through and serve.

Broccoli and Ginger: In medium-size saucepan, heat 2 cups of grain mixture with 1 cup cooked broccoli, cut in florets, 2 teaspoons grated or finely chopped ginger, 2 tablespoons water, and 1 tablespoon low-sodium soy sauce. Heat through and serve.

The Mediterranean: Mash 2 tablespoons chopped parsley or basil with 1 clove crushed garlic and 1 teaspoon grated lemon zest. Toss together with 2 cups of hot grain mixture.

Dried Cranberries and Almonds: Toss 2 cups hot grain mixture with 2 tablespoons slivered almonds, 2 tablespoons dried cranberries, and 2 tablespoons orange juice. Sprinkle with a dash of cinnamon.

Clean Cuts

Wheat berries come in soft or hard varieties, which can be used interchangeably in recipes. Soft are lower in protein and lighter in color. Hard wheat berries, usually called red winter wheat berries, are darker in color and probably should be soaked overnight (though they don't have to be). Both take a while to cook, but hard wheat berries take a bit longer (about an hour).

Wild Rice Blend

This combination of *wild rice* and brown rice has a fresh nutty taste with a hint of grassiness from the wild rice. It's called for in a number of recipes throughout the book, so make a big batch and freeze it to pull out later.

Wild Rice Blend is used in Wild Rice and Acorn Squash (see recipe later in chapter) and Wild Rice Pork Pilaf (see recipe in Chapter 18). It can also be added to any soups, such as Pumpkin and Wild Mushroom Soup or Golden Carrot Soup (see recipes in Chapter 15).

5 cups water	**⅔ cup wild rice**
⅛ tsp. sea salt	**1½ cup long grain brown rice**

Yield: 8 cups
Prep time: 5 minutes
Cook time: 1 hour
Serving size: ½ cup servings
Each serving has:
88 calories
1 g total fat
0 g saturated fat
2 g protein
18 g carbohydrate
0 g sugars
0 mg cholesterol
1 g fiber
20 mg sodium

1. In a large saucepot heat water and salt to boiling. Add wild rice. Cover and reduce heat to simmer for about 5 minutes. Add long grain brown rice. Cook for 40 minutes. Take off the heat and let rest, covered, for another 5 to 10 minutes.

2. Serve immediately plain or with a sprinkle of fresh herbs or Eating Clean Spice Blend (see recipe in Chapter 21).

Clean Meanings

Wild rice is not rice at all but the seed of a grass that grows wild in the ponds and lakes of North America. (Wild rice is the state grain of Minnesota.) Harvesting the seed is labor intensive, which explains why it is so expensive, but its strong, nutty taste means a little goes a long way.

Wild Rice and Acorn Squash

For northern Native Americans squash and wild rice was a natural combination. Here it's paired with sage, garlic, and chives. Serve this dish with a broiled chicken breast or pork tenderloin to make a hearty meal.

Yield: 3 servings
Prep time: 5 minutes
Cook time: 10 minutes (if cooking acorn squash, increase cook time by 45 minutes)
Serving size: 1 cup
Each serving has:
195 calories
4 g total fat
1 g saturated fat
4 g protein
37 g carbohydrate
2 g sugars
0 mg cholesterol
5 g fiber
32 mg sodium

2 tsp. olive oil

¼ cup red onion, diced

2 garlic cloves, peeled and crushed

2 cups Wild Rice Blend (see recipe earlier in this chapter)

1 tsp. fresh sage, finely chopped

1 TB. fresh chives or green onion, finely chopped

1 cup cooked acorn squash, cut into ½-inch pieces

⅛ tsp. ground black pepper

1. In a large skillet, heat olive oil over medium-high heat. Sauté onion and garlic in olive oil for about 2 minutes or until they begin to get soft. Add rice, sage, chives, and acorn squash.

2. Cover and heat through for 5 to 10 minutes. Stir frequently. Add 1 tablespoon water if necessary, so rice doesn't stick. Sprinkle with black pepper and serve immediately.

Variation: You can use any type of winter squash for this recipe. Try it with the Baked Butternut Squash (see recipe in Chapter 19) You can also substitute 2 cups of any type of cooked brown rice for the wild rice blend.

Clean Cuts

To cook acorn squash, peel and seed the entire vegetable. Cut into 2-inch pieces and place in roasting pan. Drizzle with 1 teaspoon olive oil and sprinkle with ⅛ teaspoon black pepper. Cover tightly with foil and bake in 375°F oven for 35 to 40 minutes.

Pineapple Brown Rice

Pineapples give this nutty brown basmati rice a sweetness you and your family will love. The ginger and green onion add some kick but are mild enough for even your little ones to enjoy.

2 cups water

1 cup pineapple juice

1½ cups brown basmati rice

½ cup fresh pineapple, diced

⅓ cup green onion, diced

1 TB. galangal (Thai ginger) or regular ginger, peeled and minced

⅛ tsp. sea salt

⅛ tsp. ground black pepper

1 TB. fresh cilantro, finely chopped (optional)

Yield: 12 servings (6 cups)
Prep time: 10 minutes
Cook time: 45 minutes
Serving size: ½ cup
Each serving has:
102 calories
1 g total fat
0 g saturated fat
2 g protein
22 g carbohydrate
3 g sugars
0 mg cholesterol
1 g fiber
26 mg sodium

1. Heat water and pineapple juice in a 4-quart pot over medium-high heat until boiling. Add rice, cover, return to a boil, then reduce heat to simmer. Cook over medium heat for 40 minutes.

2. Add pineapple, green onion, ginger, salt, pepper, and cilantro (if using). Stir, cover, and let stand 5 to 10 minutes.

Clean Cuts

Basmati is a fragrant, long grain rice native to India. Its delicate nutlike aroma and flavor has made it extremely popular in the United States, so it's easy to find. Look for it on your local grocery store shelves or at your favorite natural food store.

Barley Risotto

Mushrooms and peas make this Italian-style risotto a memorable dish. Sprinkled with a bit of grated cheese and a dash of milk it's filling enough to be a meal by itself.

Yield: 9 servings (4½ cups)
Prep time: 10 minutes
Cook time: 1 hour 15 minutes
Serving size: ½ cup
Each serving has:
120 calories
2 g total fat
1 g saturated fat
6 g protein
20 g carbohydrate
3 g sugars
0 mg cholesterol
5 g fiber
134 mg sodium

1 tsp. olive oil

½ cup onion, diced

2 garlic cloves, peeled and minced

1 (8-oz.) package sliced mushrooms (about 3 cups sliced)

1 cup whole hull-less or hulled barley

2 cups Homemade Chicken Stock (see recipe in Chapter 17) or low-sodium canned

¼ tsp. sea salt

⅛ tsp. ground black pepper

8 basil leaves, chopped

1 cup frozen peas, thawed

3 TB. Parmesan cheese, grated

¼ cup evaporated skim milk

1. Heat olive oil in a 4-quart saucepot over medium-high heat. Add onion and garlic and sauté for 5 minutes. Mix in mushrooms. Cook, covered, for about 10 minutes, stirring occasionally.

2. Add barley and brown for 1 or 2 minutes. Pour in chicken broth. Cover and bring to a boil, then reduce heat and simmer over low heat for 50 to 55 minutes. Stir in salt, pepper, basil, and peas. Cook about 10 more minutes.

3. Remove from heat and blend in cheese and evaporated milk. Serve immediately.

Variation: Most vegetables work beautifully in this risotto. If you're not sure what to use, go with the season: asparagus and onions in the spring, tomatoes and zucchini in the summer, and cauliflower and broccoli in the fall.

Clean Cuts

Polished or pearl barley is the most common type of barley you'll find in supermarkets. During processing the bran, germ, and inedible hull are stripped off. Hulled barley is the whole kernel with only the inedible hull removed. Hull-less barley, the newest type of barley on the market, is a variety in which the hull naturally falls off during harvesting. Hulled and hull-less barley take about 10 to 15 minutes longer to cook than pearl barley. If you can't find hulled or hull-less barley you can substitute pearl barley in the preceding recipe, but you'll need to adjust the cooking time accordingly.

Beans and Greens Quinoa Pilaf

Quinoa is a healthy and wholesome ancient grain native to South and Central America, so it's only fitting its deliciously nutty taste be combined with two other nutritional powerhouses, beans and greens.

Yield: 6 servings
Prep time: 5 minutes
Cook time: 25 minutes
Serving size: 1 cup
Each serving has:
189 calories
3 g total fat
0 g saturated fat
9 g protein
32 g carbohydrate
2 g sugars
0 mg cholesterol
6 g fiber
112 mg sodium

1 tsp. olive oil

½ medium onion, diced small

2 garlic cloves, peeled and minced

1 cup quinoa

1½ cups cooked red beans, drained and rinsed

8 cups fresh arugula (or other green, like spinach)

1 TB. fresh marjoram, finely chopped

2 tsp. Eating Clean Spice Blend (see recipe in Chapter 21)

¼ tsp. sea salt

¼ tsp. cracked black pepper

2 cups Roasted Vegetable Stock (see recipe in Chapter 17) or low-sodium canned

1. Heat olive oil in a large skillet over medium-high heat. Sauté onion and garlic for about 2 minutes. Add quinoa, stirring for about a minute until it starts to get toasty brown.

2. Add the rest of the ingredients. Cover and cook for 15 to 20 minutes. Quinoa will turn translucent.

3. Serve immediately with broiled chicken, fish, or steak or eat by itself for a light dinner.

Variation: You can change up the beans or the greens in this recipe, using white beans and broccoli rabe or escarole instead of the arugula and red beans.

Wholesome Habits

The ancient Incas called quinoa the "mother grain," because of its high protein content. In fact, quinoa is the only grain boasting all essential amino acids, making it a complete protein. Quinoa is also high in iron, calcium, and fiber.

Maple Veggie Mashed Potatoes

These mashed potatoes are pumped up with nutritious cauliflower and turnips. Maple syrup adds a hint of sweetness and masks the taste of the hidden vegetables. It's a surprisingly smooth, creamy, and delicious dish.

2 quarts water

½ lb. turnips, peeled and cut into 1-inch cubes

1 lb. russet or Yukon Gold potatoes (5 to 6 medium potatoes), peeled and cut into 1-inch cubes

½ lb. cauliflower (about ¼ medium-size head), cut into 1-inch cubes

2 tsp. extra-virgin olive oil

1 TB. maple syrup

½ tsp. sea salt

½ tsp. ground black pepper

½ cup unsweetened soymilk

Yield: 7 servings
Prep time: 30 minutes
Cook time: 40 minutes
Serving size: 1 cup
Each serving has:
85 calories
2 g total fat
0 g saturated fat
3 g protein
17 g carbohydrate
5 g sugars
0 mg cholesterol
3 g fiber
206 mg sodium

1. Fill a 4-quart saucepan with 2 quarts water and place over high heat. Bring to a boil. Add turnips, reduce heat to medium, and cook for 15 minutes. Add potatoes, return to a simmer, and cook another 5 minutes. Add cauliflower, return to a simmer, and cook for another 15 minutes, until all vegetables are fork tender, a total of 35 to 40 minutes.

2. Drain vegetables and mash with potato masher until mixed but still lumpy. While mashing, add olive oil, maple syrup, salt, and pepper.

3. Heat soymilk in the microwave or a small pot until hot (small bubbles will form around the edge) but not boiling (approximately 30 to 40 seconds on high).

4. Pour milk into mashed potato mixture and mash to mix. Mixture will still be slightly chunky. Serve immediately.

Clean Cuts

The high starch content of russet and Yukon Gold potatoes makes them ideal for mashing and baking. Long white potatoes, sometimes called all-purpose potatoes, will also work.

Spicy Sweet Potato Fries

These baked sweet potato fries are not for the faint of heart. They're laced with a healthy dose of spicy southwestern seasonings like smoky *chipotle pepper* and cayenne.

Yield: 4 servings
Prep time: 20 minutes
Cook time: 25 minutes
Serving size: 1 cup
Each serving has:
110 calories
1 g total fat
0 g saturated fat
2 g protein
23 g carbohydrate
5 g sugars
0 mg cholesterol
4 g fiber
208 mg sodium

1 lb. sweet potatoes, peeled and cut into long pieces ⅜-inch thick

1 tsp. olive oil

½ tsp. ground chipotle pepper

½ tsp. onion powder

½ tsp. garlic powder

¼ tsp. cayenne

¼ tsp. cumin

¼ tsp. sea salt

1. Heat oven to 450°F. Line a cookie sheet with aluminum foil and spray with cooking spray. Place potatoes in a large bowl and toss with olive oil to coat.

2. In a small bowl, mix chipotle pepper, onion powder, garlic powder, cayenne, cumin, and sea salt.

3. Sprinkle seasoning mix on potatoes and toss to coat evenly. Place potatoes on a cookie sheet in a single layer. Bake for 15 minutes. Turn potatoes with tongs (they should be beginning to brown and crisp) and bake for 10 more minutes.

4. Serve immediately.

 Clean Meanings

Chipotle peppers are jalapeños that have been dried and smoked. They are a dark, almost black, wrinkly pepper. One and a half teaspoons ground is equivalent to 1 whole chipotle pepper. Ground chipotle pepper can be found in the spice section of your grocery store. You can substitute chili powder, but it won't be as spicy or smoky.

21

Sassy Sauces and Spicy Combinations

In This Chapter

◆ Building a repertoire of clean sauces

◆ Perking up proteins with zesty spice blends and marinades

◆ Cleaning up classic sauces

Building a repertoire of homemade sauces, spice blends, and marinades is essential for managing a clean kitchen. The recipes in this chapter have much lower levels of salt and sugar than their store-bought counterparts, and since they're made from all natural ingredients, you won't have to worry about chemical additives, preservatives, or artificial colors and flavors.

You'll also be surprised at just how easy they are to make. Most recipes can be whipped together in minutes with a food processor or wire whisk. A few recipes, like Basic Clean BBQ Sauce, take longer to prepare; for these you'll want to prepare a big batch (the recipe easily doubles) to store in the refrigerator or freezer. Other recipes—such as the Eating Clean Spice Blend—may warrant a double batch simply because they become a staple in your kitchen.

Spinach Pesto

Nothing says summer like fresh pesto. In this version spinach and lemon zest lighten up traditional flavors—basil, garlic, cheese, and pine nuts—so you won't even miss the fat and calories.

Yield: ¾ cup
Prep time: 10 minutes
Serving size: 1 tablespoon
Each serving has:
51 calories
5 g total fat
1 g saturated fat
1 g protein
1 g carbohydrate
0 g sugars
2 mg cholesterol
0 g fiber
36 mg sodium

2 cups fresh baby spinach, stems removed (about 2 oz.)

12 leaves basil

4 garlic cloves, peeled and roughly chopped

3 TB. extra-virgin olive oil

¼ cup Parmesan cheese, grated

1 tsp. lemon zest

1 tsp. lemon juice

2 TB. pine nuts

2 TB. water

1. Place all ingredients in the bowl of a food processor. Process on high for about 30 seconds, scrape down the sides of the bowl with a rubber spatula, and process another 30 seconds until smooth.

2. Serve over vegetables or with pasta or meats. You can even spread on crackers.

Clean Cuts _____

Place 1 tablespoon of spinach pesto in each cube of an ice cube tray and freeze. When frozen, just pop them out, seal them in a plastic bag, and put them back in the freezer. Whenever you need pesto just pull out a cube and defrost it.

Minty Pea and Carrot Purée

This recipe breathes new life into an old-fashioned staple. Here the peas and carrots are puréed with fresh mint, lemon juice, and Parmesan cheese to produce a colorful, summery condiment that's perfect for chicken, fish, or pasta.

2 cups frozen or fresh cooked peas and carrots (1 cup peas and 1 cup carrots), thawed if frozen

1 garlic clove, peeled and sliced

3 TB. extra-virgin olive oil

¼ cup Parmesan cheese, grated

⅛ tsp. kosher salt

¼ cup Homemade Chicken Broth (see recipe in Chapter 17) or low-sodium canned

12 mint leaves (about 2 TB.)

⅛ tsp. ground black pepper

1 TB. lemon juice

2 tsp. lemon zest

Yield: 7 servings
Prep time: 10 minutes
Serving size: 2 table-spoons
Each serving has:
226 calories
12 g total fat
3 g saturated fat
20 g protein
15 g carbohydrate
1 g sugars
3 mg cholesterol
1 g fiber
378 mg sodium

1. Place all ingredients in the bowl of a food processor. Process on high for 2 minutes. Stop and scrape down the sides of the bowl with a spatula. Process another minute.

2. Serve with chicken or fish.

Clean Cuts

There are hundreds of varieties of mint that grow all over the world. The most popular are spearmint, peppermint, apple mint, and pineapple mint. Clean refreshing mint can be used in both savory and sweet dishes. Fresh is best with delicate flavors like peas, lemon, and tea; while dry is often paired with bolder tastes like red meats and tomato sauces. A little mint goes a long way. One tablespoon fresh is equivalent to one teaspoon dried.

Orange Agave Sauce

This chunky orange sauce is sweetened with agave nectar, cardamom, and cinnamon. Jalapeño pepper spices it up, but you can omit it if you can't take the heat.

Yield: ¾ cup
Prep time: 10 minutes
Cook time: 10 minutes
Serving size: 1 tablespoon
Each serving has:
51 calories
2 g total fat
0 g saturated fat
3 g protein
8 g carbohydrate
2 g sugars
0 mg cholesterol
3 g fiber
37 mg sodium

2 tsp. canola oil

1 small jalapeño, seeds and ribs removed, finely diced (be sure to use rubber gloves when handling peppers)

1 large orange, sectioned and diced

4 tsp. orange zest

½ tsp. cinnamon

¼ tsp. cardamom

3 TB. agave nectar

Pinch sea salt

1. Heat canola oil in a small saucepan over medium heat, add jalapeño pepper and cook, covered, for about 1 minute.

2. Add all remaining ingredients and simmer over medium heat for 10 minutes, stirring occasionally. Serve as a sauce on broiled meats, chicken sandwiches, and vegetables.

Wholesome Habits

Agave nectar is available in light or dark varieties. The lighter varieties have a milder taste, while the darker ones are similar to maple syrup.

Eating Clean Spice Blend

Use this easy spice blend when you want to kick up the flavor a notch. It has no salt or sugar and only a small amount of cayenne, but if you like it spicy feel free to add more. Keep it tightly sealed in a container with other spices. Use this versatile spice blend for chicken, beef, fish, vegetables, pasta, soups, and stews.

½ tsp. ground dried thyme

½ tsp. ground dried oregano

¼ tsp. cayenne

1 tsp. paprika

1 tsp. onion powder

1 tsp. dry mustard

1 tsp. garlic powder

¼ tsp. ground black pepper

½ tsp. ground cumin

Yield: 2 tablespoons
Prep time: 5 minutes
Serving size: 1 teaspoon
Each serving has:
8 calories
0 g total fat
0 g saturated fat
0 g protein
1 g carbohydrate
0 g sugars
0 mg cholesterol
0 g fiber
1 mg sodium

Mix all the spices together in a small bowl. Place in a clean dry jar, seal tightly, and store with spices. Will keep for six to eight months.

Clean Cuts

Remember that spices don't last forever. To get the freshest flavors, you should refresh your spices every six to eight months.

Clean Herb Paste

Herb pastes are a wonderful way to pump up flavor. This blend uses common herbs like parsley, basil, thyme, sage, chives, and marjoram, but, you can use almost any herb in any combination. Just go easy on strong herbs like mint and rosemary because their flavor can overpower the rest.

Yield: 1 cup
Prep time: 5 minutes
Serving size: 1 tablespoon
Each serving has:
33 calories
3 g total fat
0 g saturated fat
0 g protein
1 g carbohydrate
0 g sugars
0 mg cholesterol
0 g fiber
2 mg sodium

1 cup packed fresh parsley leaves

1 cup packed fresh basil leaves

4 TB. fresh thyme leaves

4 TB. fresh sage leaves

4 TB. fresh marjoram leaves

4 tsp. fresh chives, chopped

4 TB. extra-virgin olive oil

$\frac{1}{8}$ tsp. sea salt (optional)

$\frac{1}{8}$ tsp. ground black pepper

1. Place all ingredients in the bowl of a food processor. Process on high for about 30 seconds. If mixture looks too thick, add 1 tablespoon water.

2. Use as a marinade for meat, chicken, or fish; or toss with potatoes, vegetables, or pasta for an interesting side dish.

Clean Cuts

Herb pastes are a great way to use up old or wilted herbs. Just make a big batch, then freeze in ice cube trays for later use. If you don't want the extra fat, simply purée herbs (single or blended) with a bit of water, then freeze. You'll have clean, fresh-tasting herbs all year long.

Middle Eastern Marinade

Here we've married the flavors of India and the Middle East with a yogurt marinade tinged with Indian spices, cilantro, and garlic. It's a perfect accompaniment to grilled chicken or fish.

6 TB. nonfat Greek yogurt	**2 small garlic cloves, crushed**
2 TB. finely chopped onion	**¼ tsp. ground black pepper**
1 tsp. garam masala	**2 tsp. finely chopped fresh cilantro**
2 tsp. lemon juice	

1. Mix all ingredients together in a small bowl. Use as marinade for chicken or fish.

2. For best results marinate protein for at least an hour, preferably overnight in the refrigerator.

Wholesome Habits

Yogurt is a popular ingredient throughout Eastern Europe, the Middle East, and northern India, where it's eaten almost every day in soups, sauces, salads, and with grilled meats.

Yield: ½ cup
Prep time: 10 minutes
Serving size: 1 tablespoon
Each serving has:
9 calories
0 g total fat
0 g saturated fat
1 g protein
1 g carbohydrate
1 g sugars
0 mg cholesterol
0 g fiber
6 mg sodium

Chimichurri Sauce

Argentinean cowboys helped put this thick parsley sauce—seasoned with lemon juice and vinegar—on the map in America. Now chimichurri sauce is becoming more and more popular. Our lightened up version cuts the oil and adds pomegranate juice for a touch of sweetness.

Yield: 10 servings ⅔ cup
Prep time: 10 minutes
Serving size: 1 tablespoon
Each serving has:
20 calories
1 g total fat
0 g saturated fat
0 g protein
2 g carbohydrate
1 g sugars
0 mg cholesterol
0 g fiber
62 mg sodium

1 cup Italian flat-leaf parsley, packed

6 garlic cloves, peeled and roughly chopped

¼ tsp. sea salt

2 TB. lemon juice

1 TB. sherry vinegar

1 TB. olive oil

2 TB. fresh oregano, chopped

1 TB. red onion, finely diced

⅛ tsp. ground black pepper

2 TB. pomegranate or tart cherry juice

1. Place all ingredients in the bowl of a food processor. Blend on high for about 30 seconds or until smooth. Scrape down the sides of the bowl and process for another 10 seconds.

2. Serve on grilled chicken, fish, or steak.

Clean Cuts

Like most rustic herb sauces, chimichurri sauce has many variations and no single correct recipe. While parsley, lemon juice, and vinegar are staples, the rest of the ingredients are up for grabs. You can change it up as you like, varying the herbs and spices, adding jalapeños, or replacing the pomegranate juice with tomato or any other juice.

Clean Ketchup

This all-natural tomato-based ketchup has the same sweet-sour-spicy flavor as regular ketchup, except with a brighter taste. Nutritionally, it's also a better deal, with half the sugar and about one quarter the sodium as commercial brands. Make a big batch and save it in the fridge or freezer.

4 lb. plum tomatoes	**½ tsp. chili powder**
2 TB. finely chopped onion	**8 tsp. Sucanat**
1 garlic clove, peeled and crushed	**¼ tsp. ground allspice**
	½ tsp. sea salt
½ cup apple cider vinegar	**½ tsp. dry mustard**
1 (4–6-inch) cinnamon stick	**4 tsp. arrowroot**

Yield: 3 cups
Prep time: 25 minutes
Cook time: 40 minutes
Serving size: 1 tablespoon
Each serving has:
11 calories
0 g total fat
0 g saturated fat
0 g protein
2 g carbohydrate
2 g sugars
0 mg cholesterol
0 g fiber
51 mg sodium

1. To peel and seed tomatoes, boil 2 quarts water in a 4-quart saucepot. Fill a large bowl with cold water and ice cubes. Place whole tomatoes in boiling water for about 1 minute. Remove with tongs and place in ice bath. Let cool for 5 minutes. Take tomatoes out of ice bath, peel skin and cut in half to remove seeds.

2. Place peeled and seeded tomatoes, onion, garlic, vinegar, cinnamon stick, chili powder, Sucanat, allspice, salt, and dry mustard in a 4-quart saucepot. Cover and cook over medium-low heat (it should be gently simmering) for 25 minutes, stirring occasionally.

3. Mix arrowroot with 2 tablespoons water and add to tomato mixture. Simmer 5 more minutes (mixture will thicken slightly). Remove cinnamon stick. Pour mixture into the bowl of a food processor and process on high for 4 to 5 minutes, until very smooth, stopping occasionally to scrape down sides.

4. Place in small shallow bowls and cool for about 15 minutes in ice bath or 25 minutes on counter. Then store in refrigerator. This also freezes well.

Dirty Secrets

Typical store-bought ketchup is loaded with highly refined high-fructose corn syrup. It's also high in sodium, with one tablespoon racking up nearly 200 milligram.

Rojo Pimiento Sauce

Rojo pimiento means red pepper in Spanish and is an apt name for this mild sauce, which features roasted red peppers puréed with a dash of capers, olive oil, and garlic. Enjoy this light, refreshing, and colorful sauce with shellfish, pasta, or any type of meat.

1 large red pepper	**1 TB. sherry vinegar**
2 garlic cloves, whole, skin on	**1 tsp. capers**
1 tsp. extra-virgin olive oil	**⅛ tsp. ground black pepper**

Yield: ⅔ cup

Prep time: 15 minutes

Cook time: 25 minutes

Serving size: 1 tablespoon

Each serving has:

10 calories

1 g total fat

0 g saturated fat

0 g protein

1 g carbohydrate

1 g sugars

0 mg cholesterol

0 g fiber

9 mg sodium

---

1. Heat oven to 425°F. Spray red pepper and 2 garlic cloves (skin on) with cooking spray. Place on cookie sheet lined with aluminum foil or dry stoneware. Roast for 25 minutes. Take out and let rest for 5 minutes.

2. When pepper is cool enough to handle, peel off skin and remove seeds. Peel garlic.

3. Place red pepper, garlic, olive oil, vinegar, capers, and black pepper in the bowl of a food processor. Process on high for about 3 minutes or until sauce is smooth and creamy, stopping occasionally to scrape down the sides with a spatula. Serve warm or at room temperature over cooked chicken, fish, meat, pasta, or vegetables.

Wholesome Habits

If you have a choice between red and green peppers, go with the red. Compared to green, red peppers contain twice as much vitamin C and more than 8 times more vitamin A.

Homemade Hoisin Sauce

Hoisin is a popular Chinese sauce used in stir-fries and marinades. This clean version gives you this sauce's characteristic sweet-salty flavor but with a lot less sugar and salt than store-bought brands.

1 garlic clove, peeled and crushed	**½ small jalapeño pepper, seeded and finely chopped**
1 TB. honey	**2 TB. low-sodium soy sauce**
2 tsp. sesame seed oil	**3 tsp. rice vinegar**
2 TB. fermented black bean or soybean paste	**⅛ tsp. ground black pepper**

Yield: ½ cup
Prep time: 15 minutes
Serving size: 1 tablespoon
Each serving has:
29 calories
1 g total fat
0 g saturated fat
1 g protein
4 g carbohydrate
3 g sugars
0 g cholesterol
0 g fiber
254 mg sodium

1. In a small bowl, whisk together all ingredients until smooth.

2. Cover and refrigerate until ready to use. This sauce keeps for up to 2 weeks in the refrigerator.

Variation: If you can't find black bean paste, substitute 2 tablespoons all-natural peanut butter and add 1 tablespoon soy sauce. If that's too thick, you may want to add 1 tablespoon water.

Clean Cuts

Fermented black bean paste is available at ethnic Asian or Chinese markets. Don't confuse it with black bean sauce, which has many other ingredients added to it.

Basic Clean BBQ Sauce

This basic barbecue sauce falls into the vinegary camp, but the taste is sweet and sassy with a smoky bite, thanks to chipotle peppers. Since this recipe does take some time, make a double batch and freeze some for later.

Yield: 4 cups
Prep time: 25 minutes
Cook time: 75 minutes
Serving size: ¼ cup
Each serving has:
59 calories
2 g total fat
0 g saturated fat
1 g protein
10 g carbohydrate
6 g sugars
0 mg cholesterol
3 g fiber
112 mg sodium

12 medium tomatoes (about 1¼ lb.), cut into 1-inch pieces

2 cups onion, chopped

6 garlic cloves, peeled and minced

4 tsp. olive oil

4 TB. white or balsamic vinegar

1 tsp. ground chipotle pepper

2 TB. honey

2 TB. Sucanat

¼ tsp. ground black pepper

½ tsp. sea salt

2 tsp. low-sodium tamari

1. Heat oven to 400°F. Place tomatoes in 9×13-inch roasting pan. Drizzle with 2 teaspoons olive oil. Roast for 40 minutes.

2. Place onions and garlic in separate, smaller roasting pan. Drizzle with remaining olive oil. Roast for 10 minutes.

3. When vegetables are done, remove from the oven. Purée tomatoes in a blender and then pass the blended tomatoes through a medium-holed strainer (this will remove all the seeds and skin).

4. Return strained tomatoes to the blender, add roasted onions and garlic, vinegar, chipotle pepper, honey, Sucanat, pepper, salt, and tamari. Blend on high until smooth.

5. Pour sauce into a 4-quart saucepot. Bring to a boil over medium-high heat, then reduce heat and simmer for 20 minutes.

6. Serve warm or store in refrigerator.

Dirty Secrets _____

Many barbecue sauces use artificial ingredients like liquid smoke to give them their flavor. If you opt to buy your BBQ sauce, be sure to read the ingredients list carefully to find the cleanest one.

Part 6

Sweet Endings

Just because you're cooking clean doesn't mean you have to give up sweets. On the contrary, depriving yourself of sweet treats can cause even stronger cravings and lead to overeating. In this part, you'll find several clean sweet options.

Naturally sweet fruit is loaded with vitamins, minerals, and fiber, and is a great way to satisfy a sweet tooth. We give you plenty of ideas for preparing fruit, covering everything from Strawberry Parfait to Mango Coconut Cream.

And even though cakes, cookies, and other sweet endings should be saved for special occasions, we don't believe they should be completely eliminated from the clean lifestyle. However, they should definitely be cleaned up. The desserts in this part are light in calories, fat, and sugar, but you'd never know it by tasting them.

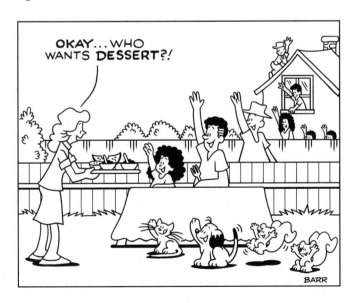

Chapter 22

Sweet Treats

In This Chapter

- ◆ Fabulous fruit desserts
- ◆ Creamy clean custards and puddings
- ◆ Incredibly light cheesecakes

Now that you've gotten used to eating whole, unprocessed, natural foods, you'll start to discover sweetness in foods you never noticed before, like snow peas, butternut squash, and beets. Even the sweetest of vegetables however, pales in comparison to fruits, which naturally contain large amounts of sugar, giving credence to the idea that fruit is nature's candy.

So, when it comes to preparing a clean dessert, fruit—alone or combined with other ingredients—is ideal for satisfying a sweet tooth. We give you a wide variety of fruit desserts to choose from—covering everything from winter pears to summer blueberries. Although most fruits are now available year round in grocery stores, you're better off buying fruit in season, when it is at its peak for ripeness and availability and prices are lowest.

Fruits have plenty to offer nutritionally, too. They're high in water, low in calories, and a good source of fiber, folate, vitamins A and C, and potassium.

You'll also find a number of cream and custard recipes in this chapter as well as a luscious Lemony Cheesecake. All of these desserts are surprisingly light and airy. Serve them to company or at a holiday party and your guests will never know they're eating clean.

The secret is simple: use all-natural ingredients and don't load up on the sugar and fat.

Use low- or nonfat dairy products. This keeps fat levels in check while still giving you a dose of dairy richness. And keep an eye on sodium. Dairy products bump up salt levels quickly.

The recipes in this chapter enable you to create fabulous everyday and special-occasion treats your family and friends are sure to *oooh* and *aaahh* over. Even more satisfying will be the fact that you've shown them that eating clean doesn't have to mean giving up your favorite treats.

Strawberry Parfait

This casual dessert is best if you wait until strawberries are in season and at their most flavorful. It's so good—and good for you—that it could easily substitute for a breakfast or afternoon snack.

½ cup plus 2 TB. nonfat, plain Greek yogurt

½ cup fresh strawberries, sliced

5 TB. Pecan Granola (see recipe in Chapter 9)

Yield: 2 servings
Prep time: 5 minutes
Serving size: 1 parfait
Each serving has:
159 calories
5 g total fat
1 g saturated fat
9 g protein
20 g carbohydrate
11 g sugars
0 mg cholesterol
2 g fiber
38 mg sodium

1. In each of 2 (10-ounce) parfait glasses, put 1 tablespoon yogurt. Layer each parfait glass with 2 tablespoons sliced strawberries, 2 tablespoons Pecan Granola, 3 tablespoons yogurt, 2 tablespoons sliced strawberries, and 1 tablespoon yogurt. Top with ½ tablespoon Pecan Granola.

2. Serve immediately or chill in refrigerator.

Clean Cuts

Strawberry season peaks in May and June. Since conventionally grown strawberries tend to be high in pesticides, it's best to buy organically grown strawberries at your local farmers' market when you can.

Pear Oatmeal Crisp

Baked pears topped with a crunchy oatmeal cinnamon crumb is a great way to end a meal. Not only does it taste delicious, the comforting aroma that fills the house will linger long after the last crumb is gone.

Yield: 4 servings
Prep time: 10 minutes
Cook time: 30 minutes
Serving size: ½ cup or ½ ramekin
Each serving has:
179 calories
6 g total fat
4 g saturated fat
3 g protein
30 g carbohydrate
11 g sugars
15 mg cholesterol
5 g fiber
3 mg sodium

2 large pears, peeled, cored, and thinly sliced

2 tsp. Sucanat

4 TB. whole wheat pastry flour

2 TB. unsalted butter, softened

6 TB. old-fashioned rolled oats

½ tsp. ground cinnamon

Pinch nutmeg

2 TB. all-natural, unsweetened apple cider

1. Heat the oven to 400°F. Spray 4 (16-ounce) ceramic ramekins or one 8×8-inch square cake pan with cooking spray. Divide sliced pears evenly among the 4 dishes or, if using cake pan, in one overlapping layer.

2. Sprinkle each ramekin with ¼ teaspoon Sucanat (1 teaspoon total).

3. In a separate small bowl mix whole wheat pastry flour, softened butter, oats, cinnamon, nutmeg, and remaining Sucanat with your fingers until small crumbs form.

4. Scatter oat mixture evenly on top of each pear ramekin, then sprinkle ½ tablespoon apple cider over top of crumbs for each dish. Bake for 30 minutes.

5. Remove from the oven. Let cool for 5 minutes. Serve warm.

Wholesome Habits

What's the difference between a crisp, a cobbler, and a crumble? Not much. They all use baked fruit as the base, but while a cobbler has a biscuit topping, a crisp generally uses oats and nuts, and a crumble is topped with flour, butter, and spices. This recipe falls into the crisp category but leaves out the nuts.

Blueberry-Kiwi Tartlet

These rustic-looking blueberry-kiwi tartlets couldn't be any simpler or more delicious. A low-fat whole wheat crust is topped with a dollop of yogurt, a drizzle of honey, and some fresh fruit. As beautiful to look at as they are to eat, you won't be able to resist them.

Crust:

1 cup white whole wheat flour

⅓ cup whole wheat pastry flour

1 TB. Sucanat

½ tsp. ground cinnamon plus more for topping

2 TB. unsalted butter, cold, sliced into four pieces

1 TB. agave nectar

¼ cup olive or canola oil

1 whole egg white

Filling:

¾ cup nonfat, plain Greek yogurt

¼ cup fresh or frozen blueberries, thawed if frozen

12 thin slices kiwi, cut in half

6 tsp. honey (optional)

Yield: 12 servings
Prep time: 10 minutes
Cook time: 10 minutes
Serving size: 1 tartlet
Each serving has:
143 calories
7 g total fat
2 g saturated fat
5 g protein
16 g carbohydrate
7 g sugars
5 mg cholesterol
2 g fiber
40 mg sodium

1. For crust: Heat the oven to 350°F. In a medium bowl mix white whole wheat flour, whole wheat pastry flour, Sucanat, and cinnamon until blended. Cut in butter with your fingers, two butter knives, or pastry blender until you form small pea-size crumbs.

2. Add agave, olive oil, and egg white and mix for about 1 minute until dough is soft and crumbly. You should be able to form a dough when mixture is pressed together with your hand.

3. Spray each muffin cup of a 12-cup muffin tin with cooking spray. Place ¼ cup dough in each cup (dough will be crumbly). Gently press dough down on bottom and about ⅓ up sides of each muffin cup with your thumb to form crust. Bake for 6 to 8 minutes. Dough will be lightly brown around the edges.

4. When crusts are cool, remove from muffin tin. Be careful as dough is very delicate and breaks easily. In each tartlet place 1 tablespoon yogurt, about 4 blueberries, 2 half slices of kiwi, and a drizzle of ½ teaspoon honey. Lightly sprinkle with cinnamon, if using.

5. Serve chilled or at room temperature.

Wholesome Habits

Blueberries are good for your brain. Studies on animals show that blueberries may protect the brain against the effects of aging by preventing memory loss and cognitive decline, so try to get a good dose of these healthful berries regularly.

Citrus-Ginger Fruit Salad

Even if you don't like grapefruit you'll love this citrus fruit salad, which also includes oranges, mint, a dash of lime, and homemade candied ginger.

Yield: 10 servings (7½ cups)
Prep time: 10 minutes
Cook time: 5 minutes
Serving size: ¾ cup
Each serving has:
60 calories
0 g total fat
0 g saturated fat
1 g protein
15 g carbohydrate
12 g sugars
0 mg cholesterol
2 g fiber
0 mg sodium

2 TB. ginger, finely chopped

½ tsp. honey

1 tsp. Sucanat

6 grapefruits, peeled and sectioned (membranes removed), plus juice

6 oranges, peeled and sectioned (membranes removed), plus juice

1 tsp. lime zest (about 1 lime)

1 TB. fresh mint, shredded or cut into *chiffonade*

1. In a small saucepan, heat ginger with honey and Sucanat until Sucanat melts and ginger softens, about 1 or 2 minutes. Set aside to cool.

2. Place grapefruits and oranges in a large bowl. You should have about 8 cups of fruit and juice. Gently mix in lime zest, fresh mint, and 1 teaspoon of cooled candied ginger. Wrap and refrigerate remaining candied ginger for another time. (It's great in Asian stir-fries or with rice. It will keep for several weeks.)

3. Keep fruit salad chilled in the refrigerator until ready to serve.

 Clean Meanings

Chiffonade is a knife skills technique in which herbs and leafy green vegetables are cut into long, thin strips. In French this word literally means "made of rags."

Fruity Melon-icious Dessert

Melon and cottage cheese are a classic combination. Our version is updated with a twist: frozen fruit is mixed right into the cheese, then topped with a sprinkle of granola. This dish is so good you can even eat it for breakfast.

⅔ cup low-fat cottage cheese

1 cup melon balls or frozen 1-inch melon cubes

1 tsp. honey

¼ tsp. ground cinnamon

2 TB. Pecan Granola (see recipe in Chapter 9)

Yield: 2 servings
Prep time: 5 minutes
Serving size: 1 cup
Each serving has:
137 calories
3 g total fat
1 g saturated fat
11 g protein
19 g carbohydrate
14 g sugars
3 mg cholesterol
1 g fiber
321 mg sodium

1. Chill melon balls in the freezer for at least a half hour or overnight. In a small bowl, stir together melon and cottage cheese. Gently stir in honey and cinnamon.

2. Scoop 1 cup of cottage cheese and fruit mixture into each of two small serving bowls. Sprinkle 1 tablespoon of Pecan Granola on each bowl. Serve chilled.

Variation: You can use nearly any type of frozen fruit for this recipe. It works great with frozen peaches, cherries, grapes, or pineapple.

Clean Cuts

Frozen fruit is a good bet when local and fresh is unavailable, because food companies pick fruit that is to be frozen when it's ripe (most conventional fruit is picked under-ripe), then freeze it quickly—sometimes the same day it's picked—ensuring a high-quality product.

Lemony Cheesecake

This lemony cheesecake is so light and fluffy you won't believe it's low in fat and calories. The secret is whipping the egg whites and then folding them back in.

Yield: 16 servings
Prep time: 25 minutes
Cook time: 75 minutes
Serving size: 1 slice
Each serving has:
191 calories
11 g total fat
5 g saturated fat
7 g protein
16 g carbohydrate
9 g sugars
51 mg cholesterol
1 g fiber
178 mg sodium

Crust:

1 cup white whole wheat flour

⅓ cup whole wheat pastry flour

1 TB. Sucanat

1 TB. agave nectar

½ tsp. cinnamon

¼ cup olive or canola oil

2 TB. unsalted butter

1 egg white

Filling:

¾ cup part-skim ricotta cheese

16 oz. low-fat cream cheese

½ cup Sucanat

¼ cup agave nectar

2 whole large eggs, separated

¾ cup low-fat evaporated milk

¼ cup lemon juice

Zest from 1 large lemon (about 1 TB.)

2 whole large eggs, separated, plus 2 egg whites

1. Heat the oven to 350°F. For crust: mix white whole wheat flour, whole wheat pastry flour, Sucanat, agave nectar, cinnamon, oil, butter, and egg white in a large bowl until just blended. Gather up dough and place in a 9½-inch springform pan, pressing down evenly with hands. Crust should be about ¼-inch thick. Bake for 10 minutes. Remove from the oven and reduce temperature to 300°F.

2. For filling: in a large bowl, add ricotta, cream cheese, Sucanat, and agave and whip by hand or using an electric mixer until light and smooth. While still mixing, add two egg yolks one at a time, evaporated milk, lemon juice, and lemon zest.

3. In a separate bowl beat four remaining egg whites until stiff peaks form, about 2 to 3 minutes, with an electric mixer. Gently fold egg whites into cream cheese mixture until just blended.

4. Place a roasting pan, ½ filled with water, on the lower rack of the oven. Lightly spray the sides of the springform pan with cooking spray. Pour cheesecake mixture into the springform pan and carefully place on the middle rack of the oven. Bake for 1 hour, until firm. Turn off the oven and let cheesecake cool inside the oven for 15 minutes without opening oven door. Place cake on wire rack until cooled to room temperature. Cover with plastic wrap and refrigerate at least two hours or overnight. Do not remove sides of springform pan until cake is cold and ready to serve.

Dirty Secrets

Our clean cheese-cake recipe has about half the fat, calories, and sugar as most store-bought varieties. So enjoy!

Almond Orange Brown Rice Pudding

Traditional rice pudding is "cleaned up" by using brown rice instead of white. Orange juice replaces some of the sugar, and almond flavored low-fat milk takes the place of cream. The result is light and low-fat but still creamy and delicious. You won't even miss the fat.

Yield: 8 servings
Prep time: 15 minutes
Cook time: 65 minutes
Serving size: ½ cup
Each serving has:
147 calories
3 g total fat
1 g saturated fat
5 g protein
26 g carbohydrate
6 g sugars
28 mg cholesterol
1 g fiber
40 mg sodium

2 TB. sliced almonds

1¾ cups water

1 cup long grain brown rice

1 whole egg

1 whole egg white

3 TB. Sucanat

½ tsp. almond extract

½ tsp. ground cinnamon

⅛ tsp. ground nutmeg

¼ cup unsweetened soymilk (optional)

Juice and zest of 1 large orange (⅓ cup juice and 1 TB. zest)

1¼ cups low-fat milk

1. Heat oven to 350°F. Place almonds in shallow pan and toast in oven for 3 to 4 minutes or until lightly brown. Set aside.

2. Bring water to a boil over medium-high heat in a 4-quart saucepot. Add rice. Reduce heat to low, cover, and simmer 40 minutes. Meanwhile, in a small bowl beat egg, egg white, Sucanat, almond extract, cinnamon, and nutmeg; set aside.

3. In a small saucepan heat 1¼ cups milk over medium heat until small bubbles begin to form around edges. Do not boil. After rice has finished cooking slowly whisk milk into egg mixture, stirring constantly.

4. Once incorporated, pour egg-milk mixture into rice pot. Gently simmer over medium heat for 10 to 15 minutes, stirring occasionally. Remove from heat and add orange juice and zest.

5. Let cool for 10 to 15 minutes. Mixture should be creamy. Sprinkle with sliced almonds. Serve warm; or cover with plastic wrap, chill in the refrigerator at least 2 hours or overnight, and serve cold. If eating cold, blend with soymilk (if using) right before serving for a creamier consistency.

Clean Cuts

If you want to speed up the cooking time for whole grains, presoak them in the allotted amount of water for a few hours prior to cooking. Then add extra water, if necessary (grains will absorb water as they sit) and cook. Presoaking can significantly cut down cooking time.

Chocolate Cherry Cream

Chocolate and cherries are a match made in heaven. Here the creaminess comes from a blend of sour cream, tofu, and yogurt. Frozen cherries keep the cream nice and cold, but fresh will work just as well.

1 oz. dark semisweet chocolate, 60–69 percent cacao

½ cup nonfat, plain Greek yogurt

¼ cup silken soft tofu

¼ cup low-fat sour cream

4 TB. chopped red sweet cherries, fresh or frozen

¼ tsp. vanilla extract

Whole cherries

Yield: 2 servings	
Prep time: 25 minutes	
Serving size: ½ cup	
Each serving has:	
136 calories	
7 g total fat	
4 g saturated fat	
8 g protein	
12 g carbohydrate	
8 g sugars	
8 mg cholesterol	
1 g fiber	
37 mg sodium	

1. Melt chocolate in a double boiler or in a glass bowl in the microwave (about 30 seconds, checking and stirring every 10 seconds to keep from burning). Set aside.

2. In a medium bowl, whisk together yogurt, tofu, and sour cream until smooth and fluffy. You may want to use electric beaters. Fold in melted chocolate, and then add chopped cherries and vanilla.

3. Divide mixture among two bowls, garnish with whole cherries, and place in the freezer 15 to 20 minutes before serving.

Variation: Almost any fresh or frozen fruit will work in this recipe. Substitute blueberries, strawberries, raspberries, or melon.

Clean Cuts

The taste of plain yogurt can vary greatly—from very tart and lemony to smooth and mild—depending on what brand you choose. Buy several brands, then taste test. Stick with the one you like.

Almond Dream Pie

This Italian-style torte highlights the flavor of almonds. Beating the egg whites first, then folding them in, keeps the pie light and airy, while sliced almonds and chocolate melted on top make for a killer presentation.

Yield: 12 servings
Prep time: 15 minutes
Cook time: 65 minutes
Serving size: 1 slice
Each serving has:
205 calories
12 g total fat
3 g saturated fat
7 g protein
18 g carbohydrate
8 g sugars
28 mg cholesterol
2 g fiber
48 mg sodium

Crust:

1 cup white whole wheat flour

⅓ cup whole wheat pastry flour

1 TB. Sucanat

1 TB. agave nectar

¼ cup olive or canola oil

2 TB. unsalted butter

½ tsp. ground cinnamon

1 whole egg white

Filling:

1 whole egg

3 TB. unsalted almond butter

8 oz. part-skim ricotta cheese

4 oz. nonfat Greek yogurt

2 TB. Sucanat

2 TB. honey

1 tsp. almond extract

⅛ tsp. ground nutmeg

2 egg whites

2 TB. sliced almonds

½ oz. dark chocolate, 60–69 percent cacao solids, grated

1. Heat the oven to 375°F. For crust: in a large bowl mix white whole wheat flour, whole wheat pastry flour, Sucanat, agave nectar, oil, butter, and cinnamon by hand or with a pastry blender until cut into uniform pea-size crumbs. Add egg white and mix gently, gathering up dough in a ball. Press into a 9½-inch deep dish pie plate. Bake crust for 5 minutes. Remove from oven and set aside to cool.

2. Reduce oven temperature to 300°F. For filling: in a large bowl, blend together whole egg, almond butter, ricotta, yogurt, Sucanat, honey, almond extract, and nutmeg. Beat until smooth. Set aside.

3. In a stand-up electric mixer, beat egg whites on high speed for 2 to 3 minutes or until stiff peaks form.

4. Gently fold egg whites into almond-ricotta mixture until incorporated. Pour into pie shell. Sprinkle pie with sliced almonds and grated chocolate. Bake for 60 minutes until firm.

5. Serve when cool or wrap and store in refrigerator overnight to be served chilled.

Wholesome Habits _____

The case for eating nuts for a healthy heart is so strong that the Food and Drug Administration recently allowed food manufacturers to say that eating 1.5 ounces of nuts along with a diet low in saturated fat and cholesterol may reduce your risk of heart disease.

Mango-Coconut Cream

Similar to a crème brulee, this mango-coconut cream is served in individual ramekins with fresh mango as a garnish. Shredded coconut adds texture. It's a perfect dessert to serve for holidays or when company is over.

Yield: 6 servings
Prep time: 10 minutes
Cook time: 80 minutes
Serving size: ½ cup
Each serving has:
131 calories
6 g total fat
4 g saturated fat
6 g protein
13 g carbohydrate
11 g sugars
77 mg cholesterol
1 g fiber
95 mg sodium

1 cup low-fat or nonfat evaporated milk

¾ cup low-fat coconut milk

1 TB. Sucanat

¼ tsp. ground nutmeg

1 tsp. arrowroot

2 TB. unsweetened grated coconut

2 whole medium eggs

2 medium egg whites

1 mango (about 12 oz. or 2 cups) peeled, pitted, and coarsely chopped

1. Heat the oven to 325°F. Combine evaporated milk and coconut milk, Sucanat, nutmeg, arrowroot, coconut, whole eggs, egg whites, and all but 2 tablespoons of mango in a blender. Process on high until mixture is smooth, about 2 minutes.

2. Divide mixture evenly among 6 (6-ounce) ramekins, sprayed with cooking spray. Place ramekins in a 9×13-inch roasting pan filled half-way with water. Carefully place in the oven and bake for 80 minutes.

3. Remove roasting pan from the oven, take ramekins out of water bath, and place on a wire rack. When cool, top each one with 1 teaspoon of reserved mango. Serve at room temperature or chill in the refrigerator and serve cold.

Wholesome Habits

Mango season runs May through September and peaks in July and August. The best mangos are firm and unblemished (they should give a little when squeezed), with a slight tropical scent. Keep in mind that the fibrousness and sweetness of a mango is determined more by variety than ripeness.

23

Clean Cakes and Cookies

In This Chapter

- ◆ Clean cakes to die for
- ◆ Nutritiously nutty cookies
- ◆ An array of antioxidant-rich chocolate treats

Who says you have to give up cookies and cakes to eat clean? Although baked goods are not meant to be an everyday indulgence, you can still enjoy these treats on occasion, with the added bonus of knowing they're healthful. Best of all, the baked goods in this chapter are just as satisfying, sweet, and delicious as conventional desserts. In fact, after trying a few of these recipes, you may even prefer them over processed cakes and cookies. I do, and so does my family.

Without white flour and refined sugar, all of these recipes supply ample amounts of fiber and are chock full of whole grains. Typically, clean cakes and cookies use less salt and sugar than conventional desserts. They also use less fat, meaning there won't be a grease stain on your napkin after eating a piece of clean cake.

Baking clean desserts does present some challenges. Most of these cakes and cookies must be stored in the refrigerator or freezer if not eaten right away, and working with 100 percent whole grain flour will take some getting used to. Since you can't usually make a direct substitution of 100 percent whole wheat flour for 100 percent all-purpose white flour without making some adjustments, you have to do some experimenting. Depending on what type of whole grain flour you use, you'll generally need to increase the liquid and/or the leavening agent.

Most cakes and cookies generously pour on the sugar, but when you start cooking clean you'll begin to appreciate natural sweeteners as something to be savored and enjoyed sparingly. We've boosted the natural sweetness of our cakes and cookies with apple, pumpkin, strawberry, and dried fruits, while coconut, nuts, and nut butters take the place of fats.

Butter, although high in fat, is included in small amounts when necessary for flavor and structure. Olive or canola oil is, of course, a better choice because it's high in heart-healthy monounsaturated fats, but it doesn't always work the same way as butter in baking.

Look at the techniques we've used to clean up some of these basic recipes, and then test out the waters with a few of your own favorites. Before you know it, you'll find yourself automatically modifying recipes to lower sugar, fat, and salt, and the results will surprise you.

Pumpkin Orange Spice Cake

Pumpkin keeps this spice cake moist and flavorful while providing a healthy dose of vitamin A. The best part is, it's so good your family and friends will never know it's clean.

1 cup honey

¾ cup canola oil

1½ cups canned pumpkin, mashed

¼ cup unsweetened applesauce

2 whole large eggs

2 whole large egg whites

2 tsp. orange zest

½ cup orange juice

1 tsp. vanilla extract

3 cups white whole wheat flour

3 tsp. baking powder

2 tsp. baking soda

½ tsp. kosher salt

½ tsp. ground allspice

1 tsp. ground cinnamon

¼ tsp. ground cloves

¼ tsp. ground nutmeg

Yield: 20 servings
Prep time: 10 minutes
Cook time: 45 minutes
Serving size: 1 piece
Each serving has:
207 calories
9 g total fat
0 g saturated fat
4 g protein
28 g carbohydrate
15 g sugars
0 mg cholesterol
3 g fiber
257 mg sodium

1. Heat the oven to 325°F. Spray a large 9×13-inch cake pan with cooking spray.

2. In a large bowl blend honey, oil, pumpkin, applesauce, eggs and egg whites, orange zest, orange juice, and vanilla until well mixed.

3. In a separate medium-size bowl whisk together flour, baking powder, baking soda, salt, allspice, cinnamon, cloves, and nutmeg.

4. Gradually add dry ingredients to wet, in two batches, gently mixing to incorporate flour. When everything is blended, pour cake batter into cake pan. Bake for 45 minutes or until cake tester comes out clean. Let cool. Cut in 20 pieces. Serve.

Clean Cuts

This cake is great for bake sales and potlucks. If you don't plan on feeding the neighborhood with it, slice it in half, wrap half of it in plastic wrap, and freeze it. It will stay fresh beautifully this way.

Apple Cinnamon Coffee Cake

Buckwheat and wheat germ give this dense coffee cake a hearty, robust flavor, while the apple and cinnamon topping adds hints of sweetness. This coffee cake is ideal as a filling breakfast treat as well as a sweet dessert.

Yield: 20 servings
Prep time: 15 minutes
Cook time: 45 minutes
Serving size: 1 piece
Each serving has:
160 calories
7 g total fat
1 g saturated fat
4 g protein
20 g carbohydrate
9 g sugars
13 mg cholesterol
2 g fiber
113 mg sodium

Crumb topping:

1 medium apple (Gala, MacIntosh, or Rome), peeled, cored, and small diced (about 1 cup)

1 TB. water

1 TB. maple syrup

¼ tsp. ground cinnamon

½ tsp. arrowroot

2 TB. whole wheat flour

1 TB. whole wheat pastry flour

½ tsp. Sucanat

1 TB. unsalted butter

Cake:

½ cup apple butter

1 whole large egg

1 whole large egg white

1 cup low-fat or nonfat buttermilk

½ cup canola oil

2 cups whole wheat flour

½ cup toasted wheat germ

¼ cup buckwheat flour

½ cup Sucanat

2 tsp. baking powder

¾ tsp. baking soda

2 tsp. ground cinnamon

1. Heat the oven to 350°F. Spray a large bundt pan or 9×13-inch cake pan with cooking spray.

2. For crumb topping: in a small saucepot over medium heat add apple, water, maple syrup, and cinnamon. Simmer for about 2 minutes until soft and apples begin to release their juice. Add arrowroot. Cook for about 1 minute until mixture thickens. Set aside to cool.

3. In a small bowl toss whole wheat flours with Sucanat and cut in butter with your fingers, a pastry blender, or two knives to make crumbs. Set aside.

4. For filling: in a large mixing bowl, beat apple butter, egg and egg white, buttermilk, and oil together. Add whole wheat flour, wheat germ, buckwheat, Sucanat, baking powder, baking soda, and cinnamon. Mix well; batter will be very thick. Let batter rest for 10 minutes. Pour into bundt pan.

5. Stir cooled apples into whole wheat crumb mixture and mix until blended. Scatter over the top of cake. Bake for 45 minutes or until cake tester comes out clean when inserted in cake.

6. Let cool. Cut into 20 slices and serve at room temperature.

Clean Cuts

Red Delicious apples aren't the best choice for this recipe because they don't soften when cooked and tend to be watery. Instead go for baking apples like Rome, MacIntosh, or Galas.

Heavenly Chocolate Cake

Coconut and applesauce keep this cake light and moist, while mini chocolate chips make it extra chocolaty. It tastes even better the next day.

Yield: 24 servings
Prep time: 15 minutes
Cook time: 25 minutes
Serving size: 1 piece
Each serving has:
165 calories
7 g total fat
3 g saturated fat
4 g protein
24 g carbohydrate
14 g sugars
9 mg cholesterol
3 g fiber
206 mg sodium

1¼ cups Sucanat

⅓ cup canola oil

¼ cup unsweetened apple-sauce

¼ cup low-fat or nonfat buttermilk

1 whole large egg

1 whole large egg white

2 tsp. vanilla extract

2 cups white whole wheat or whole wheat flour

⅔ cup spelt flour

⅔ cup plain cocoa powder (not Dutch processed)

2 tsp. baking powder

2 tsp. baking soda

½ tsp. kosher salt

½ cup unsweetened shredded coconut

½ cup mini chocolate chips

2 cups boiling water

1. Heat the oven to 350°F. Spray a 9×13-inch glass pan with cooking spray. In a large bowl mix Sucanat, oil, applesauce, buttermilk, egg and egg white, and vanilla extract until well blended.

2. In a medium bowl whisk together whole wheat flour, spelt, cocoa powder, baking powder, baking soda, salt, and coconut. Stir in chocolate chips.

3. Alternate between adding flour mixture and boiling water to the sugar mixture, beating well after each addition.

4. Pour mixture into cake pan and bake for 25 minutes or until a toothpick inserted in the center comes out clean. Remove from the oven, let cool, and cut in 24 pieces.

Wholesome Habits

Dark chocolate and cocoa are high in antioxidants called flavonoids. Studies show small amounts of dark chocolate can help reduce blood pressure and improve heart health by increasing "good" cholesterol and lowering "bad" cholesterol.

Sunflower Cookies

Mild sunflower seed butter and Sucanat produce a cookie with a slightly sweet, subtle nutty taste. These chewy, little gems are so good you won't believe they're completely wheat free. Plus, they're so easy you can whip them up in minutes.

1 cup sunflower seed butter	**1 TB. ground flaxseed**
1 cup Sucanat	**3 TB. old-fashioned rolled oats**
1 egg beaten	
1 tsp. vanilla extract	**4 tsp. roasted, salted sunflower seeds**

1. Heat the oven to 350°F. In a medium-size bowl mix sunflower seed butter, Sucanat, egg, and vanilla together. Mixture will be stiff. Add flaxseed, oats, and sunflower seeds. Let dough sit for 5 minutes.

2. Scoop a teaspoon of dough at a time, roll into 1-inch balls with your hands, and place on a cookie sheet lined with parchment paper. Flatten each cookie. Bake for about 10 to 12 minutes until lightly brown on the bottom.

Variation: If you want a lower fat vegan cookie, omit the egg. The cookies will be a bit softer but just as good.

Yield: 36 cookies
Prep time: 5 minutes
Cook time: 15 minutes
Serving size: 2 cookies
Each serving has:
141 calories
8 g total fat
1 g saturated fat
4 g protein
16 g carbohydrate
11 g sugars
16 mg cholesterol
0 g fiber
8 mg sodium

Wholesome Habits _____

If you can't find sunflower seed butter, you can use any kind of nut butter you have on hand—just change the nut to match. Peanut butter is a favorite, but almond butter will also give good results.

Strawberry Bar Cookies

These cookies are like little mini cheesecake bars, but healthier. The combination of creamy cheesecake and fresh puréed strawberries will make you swoon. Bake these cookies when sweet strawberries are in season and you're sure to draw a crowd.

Yield: 12 cookies
Prep time: 15 minutes
Cook time: 20 minutes
Serving size: 1 cookie bar
Each serving has:
152 calories
8 g total fat
2 g saturated fat
3 g protein
17 g carbohydrate
8 g sugars
9 mg cholesterol
2 g fiber
39 mg sodium

Crust:

1 cup whole wheat flour

⅓ cup whole wheat pastry flour

2 TB. Sucanat

1 TB. ground walnuts

2 TB. unsalted butter

¼ cup olive or canola oil

1 whole large egg white

Cheesecake Layer:

3 oz. low-fat cream cheese, softened

1 oz. nonfat, plain Greek yogurt

1 TB. agave nectar

Strawberry Purée:

12 strawberries, sliced

2 TB. water, divided

1 TB. agave nectar

2 tsp. arrowroot

1 TB. all-natural, fruit-sweetened strawberry spread

1. Heat the oven to 350°F. Spray a square 9×9-inch pan with cooking spray. For crust: in a medium bowl mix whole wheat flour, whole wheat pastry flour, Sucanat, walnuts, butter, oil, and egg white together to form dough. Press dough evenly into the bottom of the pan. Bake for 15 to 18 minutes. Remove from oven and set aside to cool.

2. For cheesecake layer: while crust is baking, in a small bowl whisk cream cheese, yogurt, and 1 tablespoon agave nectar until smooth and creamy.

3. For strawberry purée: heat strawberries and 1 tablespoon of water in a small saucepan for about 3 minutes. While strawberries are cooking add 1 tablespoon agave nectar and remaining tablespoon water to a small bowl and dissolve arrowroot in mixture. Add agave nectar mixture to strawberries and bring to a boil. Immediately take off the heat. Let cool for 10 minutes. Place in a food processor or mini chopper, add strawberry spread, and pulse three or four times until purée is spreadable but still chunky. Cool to room temperature.

4. When all ingredients are cool, carefully spread a thin layer of cream cheese mixture on top of whole wheat crust. Top with strawberry purée. Chill in refrigerator at least 2 hours or overnight. Cut into pieces and serve cold.

Wholesome Habits

Ruby red strawberries are loaded with vitamin C (eight strawberries contain more vitamin C than an orange), fiber, potassium, and folate. They're also rich in antioxidants, which can fight off many chronic illnesses.

Whole Wheat Chocolate Chip Cookies

When you're in the mood for chocolate chip cookies, make up a batch of these. You won't believe they're made from 100 percent whole wheat and are lower in fat, sugar, and calories compared to their traditional counterparts.

Yield: About 30 cookies
Prep time: 10 minutes
Cook time: 18 minutes
Serving size: 2 cookies
Each serving has:
140 calories
9 g total fat
3 g saturated fat
2 g protein
16 g carbohydrate
11 g sugars
20 mg cholesterol
1 g fiber
86 mg sodium

1¼ cups white whole wheat flour

½ cup oat bran

½ tsp. baking soda

¼ tsp. sea salt

3 TB. unsalted butter, softened

¼ cup canola oil

3 TB. unsweetened applesauce

1 whole large egg

1 tsp. vanilla extract

½ cup Sucanat

¾ cup semisweet chocolate chips

1. Heat the oven to 350°F. Line two baking sheets with parchment paper.

2. In a small bowl mix together flour, oat bran, baking soda, and salt. In a separate smaller bowl, beat butter until light and creamy, then add oil, applesauce, egg, vanilla, and Sucanat and beat until smooth.

3. Slowly pour wet ingredients into dry, mixing until just blended. Fold in chocolate chips. Do not over mix.

4. Spoon heaping teaspoons of dough onto baking sheets at least 1½ inches apart. Bake 15 to 17 minutes until brown around the edges. Cool on baking sheets and then transfer to wire racks to cool completely.

Wholesome Habits

This recipe uses a little bit of butter for flavor as well as for structure. Butter gives chocolate chip cookies their characteristic spread. Although our clean version will not spread as much as cookies baked with 100 percent butter, the butter does make a big difference.

Fruity Trail Mix Cookies

These incredibly moist, dense cookies are filled with almonds, dried cranberries, and healthy high-fiber grains. Just two cookies are enough to satisfy a sweet tooth and still keep fat, calories, and sugar in check—plus, they freeze beautifully.

1 cup whole wheat flour

¼ cup ground flaxseed

¾ cup oat bran

1 tsp. baking powder

¼ tsp. baking soda

¼ tsp. sea salt

2 TB. unsalted butter

3 TB. olive oil

½ cup unsalted creamy almond butter

2 TB. unsweetened applesauce

¾ cup Sucanat

1 whole large egg

⅔ cup dried cranberries

⅓ cup chopped almonds

½ cup semisweet chocolate chips

Yield: 4 dozen cookies
Prep time: 10 minutes
Cook time: 8 to 10 minutes
Serving size: 2 cookies
Each serving has:
152 calories
8 g total fat
2 g saturated fat
3 g protein
20 g carbohydrate
10 g sugars
11 mg cholesterol
2 g fiber
62 mg sodium

1. Heat the oven to 350°F. Line two baking sheets with parchment paper. In a medium-size bowl mix flour, flaxseed, oat bran, baking powder, baking soda, and salt.

2. In a large bowl, cream butter and oil. Beat almond butter, applesauce, Sucanat, and egg into butter mixture until smooth and creamy.

3. Mix flour mixture, cranberries, almonds, and chocolate chips into wet ingredients all at once, until completely incorporated.

4. Drop by heaping teaspoons onto parchment-lined baking sheets. Bake 8 to 10 minutes until golden brown and set.

Wholesome Habits

Trail mix—traditionally a mix of fruit, nuts, grains, and sometimes chocolate—got its name from hikers who carried the snack on their treks. Here trail mix morphs into a clean cookie.

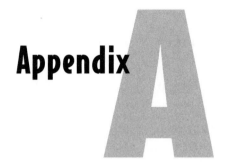

Glossary

adequate intake   A dietary intake value assigned to a nutrient when there is not enough research to support a Recommended Dietary Allowance (RDA).

aerobic activity   Any physical activity of moderate intensity which require the body to use large amounts of oxygen.

agave nectar   A natural sweetener from the Mexican agave cactus. Agave is 25 to 40 percent sweeter than table sugar (sucrose).

amaranth   A tiny grain grown in Central America that is high in protein, fiber, iron, calcium, magnesium, and folate.

amino acids   The building blocks of protein. In the body all proteins are broken down into amino acids before they can be used.

antioxidant   A type of vitamin, mineral, or phytochemical that protects the body from oxidation and, thus, the formation of free radicals. They protect us from illness and promote optimal health.

antioxidant capacity   A measure of antioxidants in a food and, thus, an indication of that food's capacity to capture free radicals.

artificial color   Man-made food dyes. Blue 1 and Green 3 are examples of colors used in some cosmetics that have been identified as potential carcinogens. Not recommended as part of a clean diet.

artificial flavor   An isolated chemical compound created in a lab by chemists or "flavorists" to enhance the flavor of a food. Not recommended as part of a clean diet.

artificial sweetener   A man-made compound meant to mimic the taste of sugar without any calories. Not recommended as part of a clean diet.

blanching   A moist heat method of cooking that involves plunging food briefly (only a few seconds) in boiling water, then chilling or "shocking" the food in ice water to stop the cooking process. A great way to prepare tender crisp vegetables.

body mass index (BMI)   A measurement of the relationship between height and weight. A BMI between 18.5 and 24.9 is an indication of a healthy weight.

bran   The protective coating around a kernel of grain; the bran is rich in B vitamins, antioxidants, and fiber.

carbohydrate   The primary energy source for the body. Carbohydrates are found in fruits, vegetables, grains, beans, and legumes.

chiffonade   A knife skill in which herbs and leafy green vegetables are cut into long thin strips. In French this word literally means "made of rags."

clean eating   Following a diet focused on whole, natural foods which are unprocessed and unrefined. It also means avoiding artificial ingredients and food additives. Typically a clean eating diet is also moderate in calories and low in fat, sugar, and salt.

coloring agent   Artificial or natural compounds that enhance the color of food. Artificial colors are not recommended as part of a clean diet.

complex carbohydrate   Nutrients made of long chains of glucose molecules; natural complex carbohydrates are starches and fiber.

convenience food   Commercially prepared processed food that is specifically designed for ease of use. Convenience foods come in boxes, bags, cans, or jars.

cruciferous vegetable   A vegetable that belongs to the cabbage family; they include broccoli, cauliflower, kale, mustard greens, collards, turnips, and rutabagas. Cruciferous vegetables are great dietary sources of nutrients such as vitamin A, potassium, folacin, and fiber, and contain phytochemicals that may help protect against cancer.

empty-calorie food   Foods that are high in calories but low in nutritive value. They are generally high in fat and sugar.

emulsifier   A substance, such as honey or mustard or the naturally-occurring lecithin in egg yolk that helps blend and stabilize a solution of oil and water-based ingredients that would otherwise separate when mixed together. Natural emulsifiers are allowed on a clean eating diet.

essential amino acid   Amino acids the body can either not make at all or can not make in adequate quantity and, thus, must get through diet. There are 9 essential amino acids the body must get from the food supply or through dietary supplements.

fiber   The indigestible part of plant matter. The average adult needs 25 to 30 grams of fiber a day.

flaxseed   Tiny seeds packed with good-for-you omega-3 fatty acids and other nutrients like magnesium, phosphorous, and thiamin. Flaxseed must be ground to be digested.

fleur de sel   A type of unrefined high-quality sea salt harvested in Brittany, France. It is produced by evaporating seawater.

food additive   Ingredients added to food to improve safety and freshness; nutritional value; or taste, texture, and appearance. They can be natural or artificial.

free radical   An unbound oxygen molecule that damages the body's cells, contributes to premature aging, and may increase risk for a number of age-related ailments and promote the development of chronic illness like certain cancers, heart disease, and arthritis.

genetically engineered animal (GE)   Animals that have had snippets of DNA from other animals, plants, or organisms inserted into their genes in order to achieve a certain outcome, such as leaner meat or disease resistance.

genetically modified organism (GMO)   Plants that have had their genes altered, typically by introducing a gene from another organism, to improve production or resist disease. Currently 70 percent of the corn and soy found in grocery stores is GMO.

germ   The seed inside a grain kernel; it's a good source of the vitamins thiamin, folacin, and vitamin E, and the minerals zinc, magnesium, and iron.

gluten   A type of protein found in rye, wheat, and barley. People who have celiac disease or are gluten-sensitive cannot eat foods containing gluten.

grass-fed beef   Meat from cattle that was raised on a diet of 100 percent grass and forage fed (no grain) with continuous access to pasture most of the season. Grass-fed meat is healthier and more nutritious than grain-fed beef.

green cuisine   Food that is both healthy and environmentally conscious. This means healthful foods that take the least amount of energy to produce. Whole, natural, clean foods are considered green.

high-fructose corn syrup   Highly refined processed sugar widely used by food manufacturers. Not recommended as part of a clean diet.

hydrogenated fat   See *trans fats*.

hypertension   Sustained elevation in blood pressure and a major risk factor for coronary heart disease or stroke. Higher than normal blood pressure is often related to many factors, including obesity, high sodium intakes, excessive alcohol consumption, and a sedentary lifestyle.

kosher salt   An unrefined coarse textured salt with no preservatives or additives. The large size crystals provide less sodium per teaspoon than finer granulated table salts due to differences in volume. Kosher salt is the preferred salt of clean eaters.

lactose intolerance   Condition in which a person is unable to digest milk and milk products because they lack the enzyme lactase to break down lactose.

locavore   Term used to describe someone who commits to buying and eating as much locally grown food as possible. How far you consider locally grown depends on the region of the country and your own personal beliefs.

millet   A mild-tasting ancient grain that's high in protein, B vitamins, iron, phosphorous, manganese, and copper.

monosodium glutamate (MSG)   Glutamic acid is a natural amino acid and its sodium salt, monosodium glutamate (MSG), is one of the most commonly used flavor enhancers. Its effect on food flavor is often referred to in Japanese as "umami" or "tastiness." However, MSG is often used as a food additive in many processed foods and should be avoided if possible.

monounsaturated fat   Fat in which the majority of the fatty acids that make up its chemical composition have only one double bond in the carbon chains, making it liquid at room temperature. Monounsaturated fats include olive, canola, and peanut oil. They are believed to have positive health benefits.

nutrient density   A measurement of a food's nutrient content compared to its calories. The more the nutrients and the fewer the calories, the higher the nutrient density.

nutrition facts panel   The part of the food label, regulated by the FDA, that contains required nutritional information for any product labeled for retail sale, including amounts for calories, fat calories, total fat, saturated fat, trans fats, cholesterol, sodium, total carbohydrates, dietary fiber, sugars, and protein.

obesity   A condition in which a person's weight is 30 percent higher than their healthy weight. People with a BMI over 30 are considered obese.

organic   Foods that are grown or raised without conventional pesticides, herbicides, synthetic fertilizers, growth hormones, antibiotics, or creating sewage sludge. Once produced, the food is minimally processed with no artificial ingredients or preservatives.

oxygen radical absorbance capacity (ORAC)   A measurement of the antioxidant capacity of foods. Certain spices, such as cinnamon; fruits, such as berries; and legumes like red beans are considered to be among those foods highest in antioxidants that can help prevent the formation of free radicals and protect the body against premature aging (see *free radical*).

partially hydrogenated fat   See *trans fats*.

percent daily value   Nutrient-intake values for a number of nutrients are developed by the FDA and are reflected as a percentage of a 2,000 calorie diet on a food label. This information is required on all food labels.

phytochemicals   Compounds that give fruits, vegetables, beans, and grains their distinct characteristics. In the body they are biologically active plant compounds that are believed to protect us from illness and promote optimal health.

preservatives   Additives that enhance shelf life, prevent foods from spoiling by protecting fats from going rancid, and protect vegetables and fruits from turning brown. They also stop the growth of mold, bacteria, and yeast. People eating a clean diet should seek to minimize the use of preservatives.

processed food   Any food that has been altered to change its physical, chemical, microbiological, or sensory properties. Not recommended as part of a clean diet.

protein   An essential dietary nutrient that is responsible for many different functions in the body, including building and maintaining lean muscle mass. Average protein intake recommendations are .8 grams per kilogram body weight per day.

quinoa   A small grain, once eaten by the ancient Incas, that is packed with protein, calcium, iron, phosphorous, B vitamins, and vitamin E.

refined flour   Flour that has had the germ and the bran removed, leaving only the endosperm. Not recommended as part of a clean diet.

refined food   Foods that have been modified to enhance shelf life or make them easier to eat or digest. They often supply a concentrated source of calories. Refined foods usually mean some part of the food has been removed, resulting in a loss of nutrients. Not recommended as part of a clean diet.

refined sugar   White table sugar, known as sucrose, which has been stripped of nutrients during processing. Not recommended as part of a clean diet.

saturated fat   Type of fat found mainly in animal foods, such as meat, butter, cheese, eggs, and dairy products. High levels are linked to increased risk for cardiovascular disease. In plant foods saturated fat is found in palm oil, palm kernel oil, and coconut oil.

sauté   To quickly cook food in a skillet or pan over direct heat, usually using a small amount of fat.

sea salt   A salt made by evaporating seawater, sea salt is considered an unrefined food.

simple carbohydrate   Simple sugars such as fructose or sucrose (see *refined sugar*).

sodium   A major mineral required by the body. Current dietary guidelines recommend no more than 2,300 milligram daily (about 1 teaspoon salt), and many health organizations suggest an adequate intake is 1500 milligram. Most Americans consume much more sodium than they need, primarily from a diet that is high in processed foods.

spelt   A nutritious whole grain in the wheat family. It can be cooked whole similar to wheat berries or ground into flour.

stabilizer   A compound used to maintain a smooth texture and uniform color and flavor in food.

standard American diet (SAD)   The eating habits of the average American. The SAD diet generally refers to a diet low in fiber, and high in animal fats and processed and fast foods; typically high in sugar, salt, fat, and artificial ingredients.

stevia   A natural licorice-tasting sweetener produced from a plant in Paraguay; it was recently approved by the FDA for use in beverages and as a tabletop sweetener.

Sucanat   Brand name of dehydrated (not evaporated) sugar cane juice. It is the least processed sugar available. Allowed on the clean eating diet.

sustainable agriculture   An agriculture method that protects and replenishes the earth's natural resources.

trans fats   Man-made fats created by adding hydrogen to liquid oils and turning them into a solid or semisolid form. On labels they are listed as "hydrogenated" or "partially hydrogenated fats." They are considered worse than saturated fats for increasing risk of heart disease. A few trans fats occur naturally in foods such as meat and other animal products, but most are man-made. Man-made trans fats are not recommended as part of a clean diet.

unrefined foods   Foods that are in their most natural state, including whole grains, whole grain flours, dried beans, legumes, and natural sweeteners like honey and maple syrup.

whole grains   All natural grains that have not been processed or refined in any way.

Five-Day Menu Plan

The meals in this menu plan should provide you with all the calories and nutrients you need while also keeping you satisfied throughout the day. Each daily menu provides 1,500 to 1,800 calories, with 20 to 25 percent of those calories coming from protein, 20 to 25 percent coming from fat, and 50 to 55 percent derived from carbohydrates. The daily sodium intake, at 1,200 to 1,650 mg sodium per day, is well below the Daily Value's 2,400 mg recommendations. In addition, you'll be getting about 30 grams of fiber or more daily. The sugar comes from added sweeteners as well as natural food sources. (To give you an idea of how this fits in, consider that nutritionists estimate the average American eats about 120 grams of only *added* sugars a day—that's not counting natural sugars found in fruits and vegetables.)

Menu Day 1

Calories: 1,665; protein: 95 grams; fat: 41 grams; sugar: 91 grams; sodium: 1,465 mg; fiber 35 grams

Breakfast

1 medium banana

1 Wild Blueberry Muffin (see recipe in Chapter 8)

1 cup skim milk

Snack

¼ cup Pecan Granola (see recipe in Chapter 9)

¾ cup nonfat, plain Greek yogurt

Lunch

1 Loaded Black Bean Burrito (see recipe in Chapter 14)

½ cup cubed cantaloupe

1 glass sparkling water

Snack

¼ cup store-bought hummus (a clean variety)

1 medium stalk celery

3 large baby carrots

Dinner

3½ oz. broiled chicken breast

¼ cup Pear Ginger Chutney (see recipe in Chapter 11)

½ cup cooked long grain brown rice

3 broccoli spears, steamed

Snack

1 TB. all-natural unsalted creamy peanut butter

1 piece rye crispbread

½ cup strawberries

Menu Day 2

Calories: 1,598; protein: 102 grams; fat: 39 grams; sugar: 93 grams; sodium: 1,100 mg; fiber: 30 grams

Breakfast

1 cup cooked oatmeal mixed with ¼ cup pumpkin, ¼ tsp. cinnamon, and ½ cup skim milk

½ cup orange juice

Snack

1 hardboiled egg

3 whole wheat crackers

Lunch

3 oz. cooked turkey breast

1 whole wheat tortilla

2 leaves lettuce

2 slices tomato

1 tsp. Dijon mustard

½ cup Apples and Nuts (see recipe in Chapter 9)

Snack

¾ cup Peaches and Cream Smoothie (see recipe in Chapter 6)

¼ cup Trail Mix (see recipe in Chapter 9)

Dinner

3 oz. roasted pork tenderloin

⅓ cup Homemade Baked Applesauce (see recipe in Chapter 11)

1 small baked sweet potato

5 asparagus spears with lemon

1 cup Acai Berry Fizzle (see recipe in Chapter 12)

Snack

3 cups air popped popcorn

1 cup skim milk

Menu Day 3

Calories: 1,515; protein: 92 grams; fat: 43 grams; sugar: 74 grams; sodium: 1,585 mg; fiber: 31 grams

Breakfast

2 Orange Buckwheat Pancakes (see recipe in Chapter 8)

½ cup Honeyed Oranges (see recipe in Chapter 11)

1 cup unsweetened soymilk

Snack

½ cup fresh blueberries

Sparkling water with a twist of lemon

Lunch

1 cup Tropical Shrimp Succotash (see recipe in Chapter 13)

½ whole wheat English muffin

2 tsp. low-fat cream cheese

1 cup unsweetened green tea

Snack

1 Banana Almond Roll Up (see recipe in Chapter 9)

Dinner

4 oz. cooked lean roast beef

1 medium baked potato

½ TB. low-fat sour cream and ½ TB. nonfat yogurt, mixed with ½ tsp. chives

½ cup Oven Roasted Brussels Sprouts (see recipe in Chapter 19)

Sparkling water with a twist of lemon

Snack

1 slice Zucchini-Carrot Bread (see recipe in Chapter 8)

½ cup unsweetened soymilk

Menu Day 4

Calories: 1,780; protein: 104 grams; fat: 44 grams; sugar: 69 grams; sodium: 1,514 mg; fiber: 45 grams

Breakfast

1 cup Kashi GoLean cereal

1 cup skim milk

1 banana

¾ cup orange juice

Snack

¼ cup oil roasted, unsalted cashew nuts

2 small stalks celery

4 slices cucumber

Lunch

1 piece Clean Broccoli Quiche (see recipe in Chapter 7)

Green salad: 1 cup iceberg lettuce, ½ cup romaine lettuce, 1 TB. chopped red onion, 1 slice tomato, 1 tsp. dried cranberries, 1 tsp. olive oil and 1 tsp. red wine vinegar, dash of sea salt, and ground black pepper

1 cup herbal tea

Snack

¼ cup low-fat cottage cheese

¼ cup diced pineapple

Dinner

3 oz. broiled tilapia

2 TB. Clean Tomato Avocado Corn Salsa (see recipe in Chapter 11)

1 cup cooked quinoa

1 cup black beans with 1 tsp. cilantro and 1 TB. nonfat Greek yogurt

Sparkling water with a twist of lime

Snack

1 cup cherries

¼ cup Pecan Granola (see recipe in Chapter 9)

Menu Day 5

Calories: 1,653; protein: 86 grams; fat: 45 grams; sugar: 88 grams; sodium: 1,598 mg; fiber: 34 grams

Breakfast

1 cup cooked oatmeal

1 cup skim milk,

¼ cup Peach Maple Jam (see recipe in Chapter 11)

2 TB. walnut pieces

¾ cup orange juice

Snack

1 oz. low-fat mozzarella cheese

¼ cup sliced strawberries

Lunch

Regal Roast Beef Sandwich (see recipe in Chapter 14)

4 baby carrots

1 medium pear

Snack

1 piece Heavenly Chocolate Cake (see recipe in Chapter 23)

1 cup unsweetened soymilk

Dinner

Asian Tofu Stir-Fry: 6 oz. of extra-firm tofu, 1 cup mixed steamed vegetables, 1 tsp. low sodium tamari, 1 TB. water, ½ tsp. each ginger and garlic, and a dash of hot sauce. Sauté in pan with 1 tsp. sesame seed oil.

¾ cup brown short grain rice

1 cup green tea

Snack

3 Date Coconut Crisps (see recipe in Chapter 9)

Sparkling water with a twist of lemon

Index